HOME REMEDIES

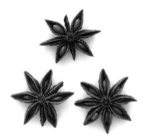

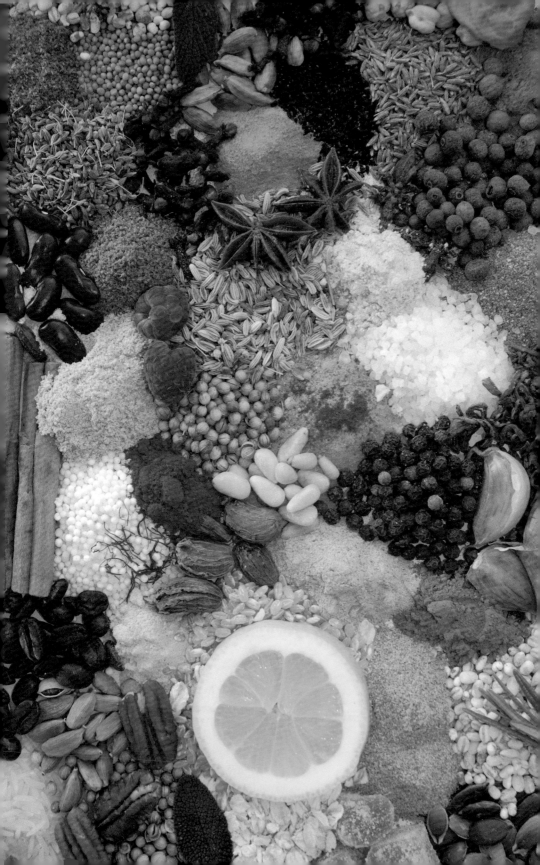

HOME REMEDIES

How to Use Kitchen Staples to Treat Common Ailments

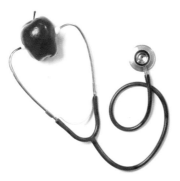

JULIE BRUTON-SEAL
MATTHEW SEAL

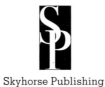

Skyhorse Publishing

Skyhorse Publishing books may be purchased in bulk at special discounts for sales
promotion, corporate gifts, fund-raising, or educational purposes. Special editions
can also be created to specifications. For details, contact the Special Sales Department,
Skyhorse Publishing, 307 West 36th Street, 11th Floor, New York, NY 10018 or
info@skyhorsepublishing.com.

Skyhorse® and Skyhorse Publishing® are registered trademarks of Skyhorse Publishing, Inc.®,
a Delaware corporation.

Visit our website at www.skyhorsepublishing.com.

10 9 8 7 6 5 4 3 2 1

Library of Congress Cataloging-in-Publication Data is available on file.

Cover design by Mona Lin

Designed and typeset by Julie Bruton-Seal and Matthew Seal
Photographs by Julie Bruton-Seal

Print ISBN: 978-1-5107-5405-8
Ebook ISBN: 978-1-5107-5705-9

Printed in China

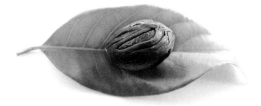

Please note:
The information in *Home Remedies* is compiled from a blend of historical and
modern scientific sources, from folklore and personal experience. It is not intended to
replace the professional advice and care of a qualified herbal or medical practitioner.
Do not attempt to self-diagnose or self-prescribe for serious long-term problems without first consulting a qualified professional. Heed the cautions given, and if already
taking prescribed medicines or if you are pregnant, seek professional advice before
using herbal remedies.

Contents

Preface

This book is our second collaboration with Merlin Unwin Books, following *Hedgerow Medicine* in 2008. Once more we are hugely grateful to Merlin, Karen and Jo, who have trusted us to put the positive case for the safe medicinal use of tea, sugar, sage and the many other kitchen products we examine.

As before, Julie was the expert herbalist and photographer, Matthew the editor and camera bag carrier, while we shared all the writing and idea-hatching. We have maintained the format and layout of the previous book, but have expanded the number of chapters. A reference list by ailment (red-bordered pages from p189) is a new addition.

People across four continents let us loose to photograph their kitchens, and we thank in particular Paula Stone, Karin Haile, Lyndall Strazdins and Tim Edmondson, Les Bartlett, Sara and Andrew Butcher, and Jenny Carvill.

Thanks also go to Julie's mother Jen Bartlett for the author photo, and Denise Burcher and Karen Palmer for their help in various ways.

Susie Allan, Julie's 'big sister' in Kenya, organised a trip to tea and coffee plantations with her partner Brian Williams. We thank all at Kamundu Estate (Sasini) and Karirana Estate who showed us around on a wet day and found us ripe coffee beans to photograph, followed by misty tea fields, respectively.

Said Mohammed and his assistant James guided us through a prolific spice garden in Zanzibar and found us specimens from all-spice to ylang-ylang. Thomas Tomichen was equally helpful in southern India.

Herbalist and friend Christine Herbert again provided invaluable assistance in checking the text, and looked after some of Julie's patients while we were away on photographic trips. Her partner Mark Naylor grew many of the vegetables featured on these pages.

We acknowledge that the opinions expressed here are our own, and we take responsibility for them. Sources are referenced in the notes to the text section, and we thank copyright holders for permission to include extracts from their work. If we have overlooked or been unable to locate any copyright owner we will gladly add details in a later edition.

We thank John Ambrose and the John Innes Foundation Collection of Rare Botanical Books, Norwich for permission to photograph and read classic herbal works in a splendid library just down the road from us. We are also grateful to the British Library, Wellcome Library and Norfolk Record Office for their unfailing help, and for still being there.

Julie Bruton-Seal & Matthew Seal
Ashwellthorpe, Norfolk   May 2010

A note on the 2019 reprint
We have taken this opportunity to update data wherever possible, revise the scientific names of plants according to the Kew *Plant-List*, change a number of the photographs, bring the resources and reading lists up to date, and generally refresh the book.

Julie Bruton-Seal & Matthew Seal
Ashwellthorpe, Norfolk   June 2019

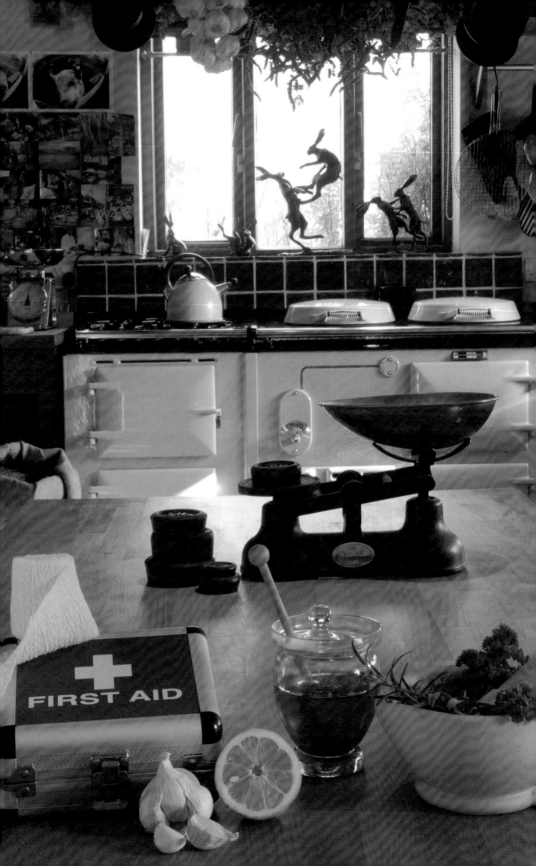

Introduction

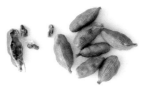

In times past, kitchen medicine was practised by every housewife. She may not have used the term or even thought about it much, but she would have learned how to treat her family for everyday ailments and minor emergencies with what she had to hand.

Doctors were expensive, and our ancestors had to be more self-reliant in their healthcare. Matthew's mother would recall England in the 1920s, when going to the doctor meant a fee of a shilling, a hefty charge; as a child she was sent to the corner shop for 'a ha'p'orth of ipecacuanha'. Our grandmothers used laundry blue for wasp stings and bicarb for upset tummies, and hot lemon and honey drinks for colds. Chicken soup was a cure-all, and if in doubt, a nice cup of tea was just the thing.

We think it is time to revive this disappearing tradition of using your pantry as your pharmacy. Indeed, the kitchen is where you are most likely to need first aid. For a domestic space that can still claim to be the centre of family life – of cooking, warmth, storage and conviviality – the kitchen can be a rather dangerous place. The Royal Society for the Prevention of Accidents in 2017 reported 2.7 million people in Britain went to A&E departments after accidents in the home, and 5,000 people died. Most of these mishaps were in the kitchen or on the stairs, often involving the very young or the elderly.

By contrast, in British industry in a typical year there are some 550,000 non-fatal accidents notified. Clearly, this reflects the different age populations and regulation of

conditions in the workplace and at home, but the discrepancy in the figures is telling. We do need to be better informed on first aid matters and take more self-responsibility for health and safety in our own home.

What can the individual do? We believe it is part of what might be called a 'medicinal intelligence' to seek to become more aware of the potential health value of food and food-related products that are stored but often ignored in our kitchens.

You might imagine this is a flourishing field of study, but it has been neglected. It falls beneath the eye level of orthodox medicine and orthodox herbalism alike, and while part of family lore and generically within folk medicine, linking the two familiar concepts 'kitchen' and 'medicine' is rarely done. An exception is Jill Davies, one of Julie's herbal medicine teachers, a strong proponent of kitchen pharmacy and self-healing, who has done much to promote this awareness.

The leading books in this small field were published some sixty and thirty years ago (respectively Ben Charles Harris, *Kitchen Medicines*, 1961 and Rose Elliot & Carlo de Paoli, *Kitchen Pharmacy*, 1991). These remain excellent of their time, but neither has the eclectic and illustration-rich approach we adopt. The most comparable newish book to our own, the late Christopher Hedley & Non Shaw's *Herbal Remedies* (1996), is hard to come by and should be better known.

We'd like to share with you our curiosity about the remarkable, exotic treasures sitting in our kitchens and pantries, which, in the last authors' words, 'would have been the envy of an 18th-century apothecary'. It has been especially fascinating to learn at first hand more of the history of spices, where things come from, how they grow and how familar products are made.

We believe, with Hedley & Shaw, that 'No matter what ailment we may suffer from, we can always do something ourselves to enhance our well-being.' Our *Backyard Medicine* was a guide to medicinal plants and weeds you can gather for yourself outdoors; now *Home Remedies* is a guide to health resources indoors sitting on your kitchen shelf.

We believe a working knowledge of kitchen medicine is a valuable life skill acquisition. There is usually something in your fridge or pantry that will meet your medicinal need – a great asset in the middle of the night or on a public holiday when the chemists are shut. It's also going to save you money.

You may be surprised to see items like coffee, tea and white rice in our coverage, presuming a contemporary herbalist would be against them. What we are actually against is food puritanism and prescriptiveness: everybody has different needs, constitutions and starting points. It is up to each of us how we use these potential gifts from our kitchen shelves. Some people tolerate a bell pepper, others a habañero, but if used appropriately both earn their keep as food and (we argue) medicine.

Kitchen medicines are by definition safe, or we wouldn't have the products in our pantries. The continuum food / medicine / poison is largely a matter of dosage, and too much of anything can cause problems –

nothing could seem safer than water and yet drinking too much too quickly can be fatal.

The intensity of taste is a practical guide to dosage in medicine as it is with cooking, with blander things like cabbage being classed as vegetables and strong, intense flavours like cloves being called spices and used sparingly. Kitchen medicines generally taste good, as they are made from things we eat anyway. Moderation and balance are the goal, if hard to achieve, and you can always say no. As St Augustine wrote: 'Complete abstinence is easier than perfect moderation.'

We give cautions as necessary and propose moderate dosages. We are deliberately not too specific in our recipes, preferring you to follow the general idea of the remedy and find your own comfort level with it. Use lower quantities for children and older people, and for anyone who is weak or sensitive.

In general do not self-diagnose for other than straightforward conditions, and please consult a medical or herbal practitioner if you are pregnant, taking other medication or are in any way unsure of your ground. We don't want you to be a statistic of accidents at home from using our recipes!

Note: a teaspoon is about 5ml and a tablespoon three times larger, at 15ml. A cup is a regular kitchen cup of about 250ml or 8 fl oz.

We hope our book will inspire you to look again at everyday items in your kitchen and pantry. Whether used as food, spices, herbs or condiments, or even for cleaning, many are potentially valuable for first aid and to treat common ailments.

The ingredients

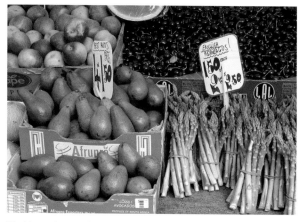

Weekly markets and
farmers' markets are
good places to shop
for your fresh fruit and
vegetables

We have chosen 60 products,
many of which are probably
already in your kitchen. Our
list subdivides into 25 herbs
and spices, 26 vegetables and
fruits and 9 others (such as
water, vinegar and salt). Some
items overlap categories (eg
chilli is both vegetable and
spice), but around half are
perishables and the rest stored
goods you might keep for
years. All have a role in your
home medicine chest.

My Dear Sir,
A thousand thanks
for the Banana, it
arrived quite safe
and I am delighted to
have an opportunity
of seeing that
most beautiful and
curious Fruit. It is
the admiration of
everybody and has
been feasted upon
at dinner today
according to the
directions.

– From a letter by
William Spencer
Cavendish, 6th Duke
of Devonshire, 1834.
By 1836, the 'dwarf
Cavendish' banana
had been developed
at Chatsworth. It
is now the leading
banana cultivar
worldwide.

Buying fruits and vegetables

You don't need to change the
way you shop, but there are a few
things to consider when using
foods as medicines. First, they
should be as fresh as possible, and
free from chemicals.

Anything you can grow yourself
is not only the freshest available
but you also know exactly
what it is or what went into it.
Organically grown foods should
be the next best, but air miles
count: sometimes you must choose
between local and really fresh or
something organically certified but
shipped halfway around the world
and thus more costly to you and to
the environment.

Many areas have local organic
box delivery schemes, and you
can find these online. Markets,
farmers' markets and farm shops
are another source of cheaper,
fresher produce than you may find
in a large food store.

Buying dried herbs and spices

The small jars normally sold
in supermarkets are not really
economical. Buy bigger bags from
an Asian grocer's or a herbalist
– these will often be fresher and
better quality as well as cheaper.

We give contacts for some
excellent British herbal suppliers
(p204): these resource professional
herbalists but also have active
retail and mail order facilities.

Storing dried herbs and spices

Herbs and spices are best stored
in glass jars and in a cool place. If
your jar is clear glass, keep it in the
dark, as light will fade and age the

contents. Brown or blue glass jars help protect contents from light.

Whole dried herbs will usually keep for about a year, but powders usually less than that. Saying that, though, we have found that stored ground black or white pepper is still potent after several years. Whole seeds or spices, like coriander or cloves, often last well (some accompany ancient Egyptian mummies).

Smell and taste will fade with time, as do medicinal properties, especially if the active agent is a volatile oil. To check if something is still good, smell it and taste it. If in doubt, put old herbs or spices on your compost and replace them with even better-quality ones. Anything that has languished on pantry shelves for years is unlikely to have much medicinal power.

Storing other dried goods

This is the easy part: your tea, coffee, bicarb (baking soda), salt, honey, sugar or vinegar, say, are purchased in packets or bottles that can be stored as they are. Once you make ghee it can last indefinitely. Some of our recipes simply involve adding herbs to honey or vinegar, while tinctures are easily made from almost any type of alcohol (see overleaf).

Make your own 'receipt' book

We don't know anything about Sophia Baillie (right), but her two-hundred-year-old receipt book has been preserved, as have many hundreds more in archives. Her cordial sounds a tasty addition to external rheumatism treatments, and the formula was probably passed down in her family. We can do the same for our children – perhaps online, with photos.

A cordial for rheumatism
Taken from the handwritten receipt book of Sophia Baillie, 1819 (courtesy of Norfolk Record Office)

Put into a quart bottle, 3 table spoonfuls of scraped ginger, 1 tea spoonful of made mustard, and 4 large wine glasses of gin. Fill up the bottle with ale, sweeten it with brown sugar, & take two tea spoonfuls in a cup of warm water every night & morning.

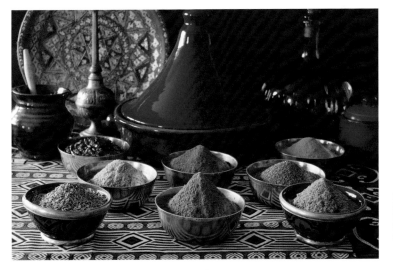

Spices from an Oriental grocery are often fresher and cheaper than those from a supermarket

Using kitchen medicines

The ingredients discussed in this book are all foods (or food-related) as well as medicines, and one of the best ways to use them medicinally is as foods. Once you learn more about each ingredient and how it affects the body, you'll be able to adjust your cooking to the health needs of the people eating it.

In addition, many food ingredients can be used in other ways – as skin creams, poultices or baths, for example. This section gives a quick summary of different ways you can prepare them as medicines. Every family has its favourite remedies for colds and common ailments, and we hope we will inspire you to experiment with new ideas and develop your own recipes for medicines you can make at home.

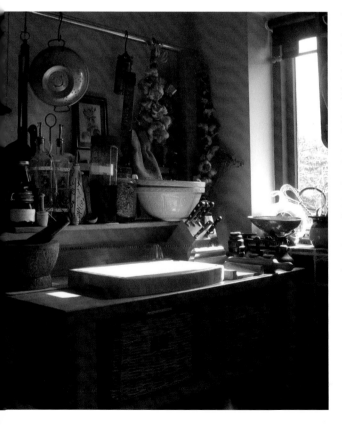

The good news is you don't need any special equipment for making your own kitchen medicines.

Kitchen basics like a teapot, measuring jugs, saucepans and a blender are all useful, as are jam-making supplies. Treat yourself to a mortar and pestle or electric grinder if you don't already have one.

You'll need jars and bottles, and labels for these. Use a notebook to write down your experiences and the quantities used as a record for yourself, so you can repeat your successes. Who knows, it could become a future family heirloom like the receipt books of old!

Drying herbs
You may grow your own culinary herbs, and want to dry them for winter use. To dry herbs, tie them in small bundles and hang these upside down from the rafters or a laundry airer, or spread the herbs

on a sheet of brown paper or a screen. (Avoid using newspaper as the inks can have toxic chemicals.)

You can easily make your own drying screen by stapling some mosquito netting or other open-weave fabric to a wooden frame. This is ideal, as the air can circulate around the plant, and yet you won't lose any small flowers or leaves that are loose. Generally, plants are best dried out of the sun. An airing cupboard works well, especially in damp weather. Don't dry herbs in the microwave, though, as it could alter the plant's chemistry.

Once the plant is crisply dry, you can discard any larger stalks. Whole leaves and flowers will keep best, but if they are large you may want to crumble them so they take up less space. They will be easier to measure for teas etc if they are crumbled before use.

Teas: infusions and decoctions

The simplest way to make a plant extract is with hot water. Either fresh or dried herbs can be used, though don't forget that a dried herb is already concentrated and you need far less.

An **infusion,** where hot water is poured over the herb and left to steep for several minutes, is the usual method for a tea of leaves, flowers and aromatic seeds.

A **decoction**, where the herb is simmered or boiled in water for

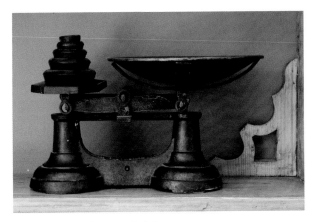

some time, is often needed for large seeds and bark, which are tougher and have more protective layers. Infusions and decoctions can also be used as mouthwashes, gargles, eyebaths, fomentations and douches, or added to baths.

Tinctures

While the term tincture can refer to any liquid extract of a plant, what is usually meant is an alcohol and water extract. Many plant constituents dissolve more easily in a mixture of alcohol and water than in pure water. An additional advantage is that alcohol is a preservative, allowing the extract to be stored for several years.

For making your own tinctures, vodka is one of the best alcohols to use as it has no flavour of its own, and allows the taste of the herbs to come through. Whisky, brandy or rum work well too, if you like their flavour. Wine can be used, especially for dried herbs, but will not have as long a shelf life.

Joy, temperance and repose,/
Slam the door on the doctor's nose.
– Von Logau (c. 1654)

To make a tincture, you simply fill a jar with the herbs and top up with alcohol, or you can put the whole lot in the blender first. The mixture is then kept out of the light for anything from a day to a month to infuse before being strained, bottled and labelled.

Tinctures are convenient to store and to take. We find amber or blue glass jars best for keeping, although clear bottles will let you enjoy the colours of your tinctures. Store them in a cool place. Kept properly, most tinctures have a shelf life of around five years. They are rapidly absorbed into the bloodstream, and alcohol makes the preparation more heating and dispersing in its effect.

Vinegars

Herb and spice vinegars can be used in salad dressings and for cooking. They are also a good addition to the bath or for rinsing hair, as the acetic acid of the vinegar helps restore the natural protective acidic pH of the body's exterior. Cider vinegar is a remedy for colds and other viruses, so it is a good solvent for herbs taken for these conditions.

Herbal honeys

Honey has natural antibiotic and antiseptic properties, and makes an excellent and quickly absorbed vehicle for medicines to fight infection. Apply externally to wounds and burns. Locally made honey can help prevent hayfever attacks.

Oxymels

An oxymel is a preparation of honey and vinegar. Oxymels were once popular as cordials, both in Middle Eastern and European traditions. They are particularly good for cold and 'flu remedies. Honey can be added to a herb-infused vinegar, or an infused honey can be used as well.

Electuaries

These are made by stirring powdered dried herbs into honey or a syrup to make a paste. Electuaries are good as children's remedies, and are often used to soothe the digestive tract. This is also a good way to prepare hay fever remedies and tonic herbs.

Syrups

Syrups are usually made by boiling the herb with sugar and water. The sugar acts as a preservative, and can help extract the plant material. Syrups generally keep well, especially the thicker ones containing more sugar, as long as they are stored in sterilised bottles. Syrups are particularly suitable for children because of their sweet taste, and are generally soothing.

Infused oils

Oil is mostly used to make preparations for external use on the skin, but herbal infused oils can equally well be taken internally. Like vinegars, they work well in home-made salad dressings and in cooking.

We prefer extra virgin olive oil as a base, as it does not go rancid like many polyunsaturated oils do. Other oils, such as coconut and sesame, may be chosen because of their individual characteristics.

Infused oils are often called macerated oils, and should not be confused with essential oils, which are aromatic oils isolated by distilling plant material and are generally not taken internally.

Ointments or salves

Ointments or salves are rubbed onto the skin. The simplest ointments are made by adding beeswax to an infused oil and heating until the beeswax has melted. Use about 25g of wax per 300ml of oil. The more wax used, the stiffer the ointment. You may want to vary the amount, depending on the climate, with more wax needed in hotter climates or weather.

Ointments made this way have a very good shelf life. They absorb well, while providing a protective layer on top of the skin.

Ointments can also be made with animal fats, such as lard, butter or ghee, or from hard plant fats such as coconut oil and cocoa butter.

Skin creams and lotions

Creams and lotions are made by mixing a water-based preparation with an oil-based one, to produce an emulsion. Dairy cream can be used for fresh products, as it is a natural emulsion.

Creams and lotions are absorbed into the skin more rapidly than ointments, and are less greasy but have the disadvantage of not keeping as well. Essential oils can be added to help preserve them.

Poultices

The simplest poultice is mashed fresh herb put onto the skin, as when you crush a cabbage leaf and apply it to an insect sting. Poultices can be made from fresh juice mixed with a powder such as cornflour or oatmeal, or from a dried herb or spice moistened with hot water or vinegar.

Change the poultice every few hours and keep it in place with a bandage or sticking plaster.

Fomentations or compresses

A fomentation or compress is an infusion or a decoction applied externally. Simply soak a flannel or bandage in the warm or cold liquid, and apply.

Hot fomentations are used to disperse and clear, and are good for conditions as varied as backache, joint pain, boils and acne. Hot fomentations need to be refreshed frequently once they cool down.

Cold fomentations can be used for inflammation or for headaches. Alternating hot and cold fomentations works well for sprains and other injuries.

Embrocations or liniments

Embrocations or liniments are used in massage, with the herbs in an oil or alcohol base or a mixture of the two. Absorbed quickly through the skin, they can readily relieve muscle tension, pain and inflammation, and speed the healing of injuries.

Baths

Kitchen medicines can be added conveniently to the bath by tying a sock or cloth full of dried or fresh herb to the hot tap as you run the water, or by adding a few cups of an infusion or decoction into the bath. Herbal vinegars and oils can also be added to hot baths.

Besides full baths, hand and foot baths can be very effective treatments, as can sitz or hip baths where only your bottom is in the water.

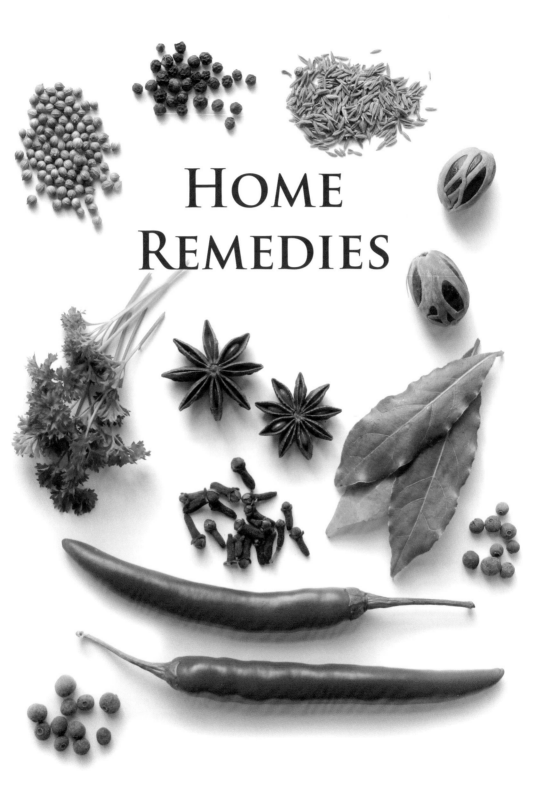

HOME
REMEDIES

Allspice

Pimenta dioica syn. *P. officinalis*

Pimento, Jamaica pepper

Allspice is one of the few spices from the New World. It is antiseptic and settles the stomach, relieving flatulence and indigestion, while used externally it has an anaesthetic effect on toothache as well as muscular and rheumatic aches and pains. An allspice tea clears the head, helps in concentration and improves metabolism.

Myrtaceae
Myrtle family

Description: A tropical tree growing to 12m (37ft); it bears panicles of fragrant white flowers, which are followed by the berries.

Distribution: Native to the Caribbean, south-ern Mexico and Central America, extensively cultivated in Jamaica and introduced to the Pacific islands.

Related species: *P. racemosa* syn. *P. acris* was once important as the source of bay rum, used in aftershaves and hair dressings.

Parts used: Berries. The fresh leaves are used in infusions, and for distilling an essen-tial oil.

... a sweet-scented Jamaica pepper or allspice.
– Ray (1693)

... the only spice whose production is confined to the New World.
– Davidson (1999)

It sometimes surprises people that allspice is not a mixture of several ground spices but is in fact the dried, immature red–brown fruit of a beautiful evergreen Caribbean tree. It would not be the first confusion this spice has caused.

First imported to Europe by the Spanish in the sixteenth century, allspice was known to herbalists but not given its enduring English name until the botanist John Ray coined it in 1693.

Ray chose the name after comparing the flavour to a combination of cloves, cinnamon and nutmeg. Other people say they get a reminder of juniper or black pepper; we think most of cloves and pepper.

Early Spanish traders detected a resemblance to pepper and called the Jamaican fruit a pimiento, from Spanish *pimienta* or peppercorn. Confusion arises because the New World capsicums and chillies were also known as peppers, and are often called pimientos. Pimentos

and pimientos are still often mistaken for each other.

Pimento essential oil is distilled from the leaves of the tree, and is used in antioxidants, anaesthetics and muscle relaxants.

Allspice was an official plant of the *British Pharmacopoeia* for nearly two hundred years, from 1721 to 1914, but is less used in herbal medicine nowadays.

Use allspice for...
You may already have a supply of allspice to flavour fruit drinks or mulled wine. We like it in hot spiced apple juice in wintertime.

Commercially allspice has been an ingredient in the liqueurs Benedictine and Chartreuse and the Caribbean pimento liqueur. It is also a good pickling agent.

Allspice is an aromatic digestive stimulant, in which it resembles cloves. Both spices share an anaesthetic quality. Allspice has a mild numbing effect, and is a

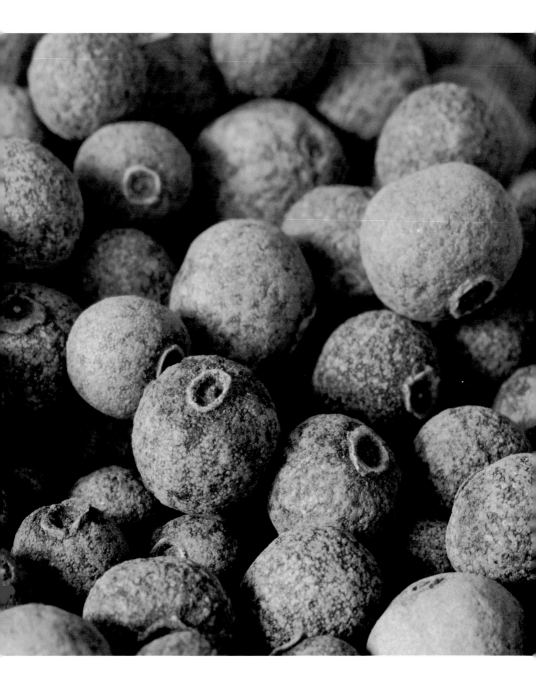

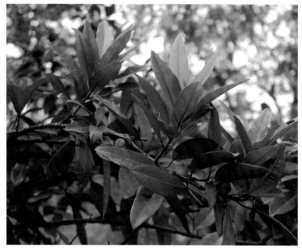
Allspice growing in Singapore

bittersweet aroma. Eugenol has been found to boost the action of the digestive enzyme trypsin, which serves to settle the stomach. Allspice is certainly used in rich Caribbean stews for this purpose, as well as for its flavour.

Allspice works best when crushed, releasing its distinctive aroma. The powder does not last as well as the dried berries, so for medicinal use we suggest keeping the berries whole in an airtight glass jar, preferably out of the light, and grinding them as needed.

Allspice paste can be used externally in a plaster or poultice to bring relief to rheumatic, arthritic or muscular pain.

Another use favoured by herbalists is as a tonic, drunk to improve metabolic processes in the body overall.

good alternative to cloves as a mouthwash or to pack against an aching tooth.

The similarity arises from the fact that both spices contain an appreciable amount of the oil eugenol, which lends the evocative

Allspice tea
- flatulence
- indigestion
- digestion
- fungal infections
- poor circulation
- menopause
- clears the head

Allspice mouthwash
- bad breath
- gum problems
- toothache

Allspice paste
- insect bites

Caution: Do not take allspice medicinally during pregnancy. Prolonged exposure can irritate delicate skins, creating a kind of contact dermatitis, and if you find any redness on the skin when using allspice externally, it is best to stop.

Allspice tea
Use ½ teaspoon of crushed **allspice berries** to a cup of **boiling water** and allow to infuse for several minutes. It is a lovely warming digestive drink either before or after meals.

The cooled tea can be put in a spray bottle for use as an air freshener. It is antiseptic, and can be sprayed onto fungal infections or used to freshen kitchen surfaces.

Allspice mouthwash
Make a double-strength tea, using a teaspoon of crushed **allspice berries** to a cup of **boiling water** and allow to infuse for 15 minutes. Strain and use as a mouthwash. Keeps for several days in the fridge.

Allspice paste
Make a paste with **allspice powder** and a little **water**. Apply to insect bites for topical relief.

Almond

Prunus dulcis syn. *P. amygdalus* syn. *Amygdalus communis*; var. *dulcis* (sweet almond); var. *amara* (bitter almond)

Almonds have been grown since prehistoric times, and are the most important nut cultivated commercially. Bitter almonds provide the characteristic flavour of marzipan, while sweet almonds are mild in flavour and make one of the best non-dairy milks. Almonds are alkalising and nutritious, and soothe dry coughs and inflamed intestines.

Almonds are an ancient food and medicine deriving from central and west Asia, and most associated with the Mediterranean and similar climatic zones. A jar of almond nuts was found in the tomb of Pharaoh Tutankhamun (died about 1325 BC), and scholars maintain that the Aaron's rod that flowered in the Book of Numbers of the Bible was an almond.

Interestingly, in terms of the botany of the tree, one part of the Aaron tradition states that the rod flowered on both sides, one sweet and one bitter, interpreted as one for the way of righteousness offered to the Israelites and one for its denial.

As befits a long association with man, almond has borne multiple scientific names in the past. It seems now to have settled on a simple *Prunus dulcis*. But note that the old split between sweet (var. *dulcis*) and bitter almond (var. *amara*) remains, and if the two are still twins they are definitely non-identical.

There is a small visual difference in the fruit, with the sweet almond somewhat larger, but the blossoms give it away: those of the sweet almond are usually fluffy and white, with some red at the centre, while those of its bitter twin are predominantly pink.

Both nuts have a good proportion of fine almond oil (around 50% by weight) and protein (around 20%), and generous helpings of vitamins and minerals, but what gives the

Rosaceae
Rose family

Description: A small deciduous tree. Beautiful white or pale pink flowers are borne in spring, followed by leathery fruit containing the large nut.

Distribution: Native to the Middle East, now grown worldwide.

Related species: Other species in the genus include apricot (*P. armeniaca*) and sweet cherry (*P. avium*) as well as peaches, nectarines and plums.

Parts used: Nuts, oil.

Almond, from Woodville's *Medical Botany* (1790–3)

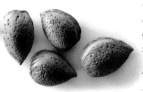

bitter almond its name, aroma and taste is the presence (2–4%) of amygdalin, a toxic glycoside.

This becomes the poison prussic acid (hydrogen cyanide) when water is added and bitter almonds are crushed, but processing and heating render it harmless.

The abbreviation FFPA (free from prussic acid) is applied to the processed almonds. The sale of bitter almonds is now prohibited in the US, but all the same this is the form most used for almond essence, marzipan, confectionery, ice cream and other commercial uses (completely safely). Sweet almonds are the nuts sold to eat, and are the main source of the almond oil used in massage, skincare products and cosmetics as well as medicinally.

The link between almonds and the brain is intriguing. The old botanical name for almond is *amygdala* (corrupted in time and across languages into 'almond'), and the same name has been given to two almond-shaped parts of the brain. These brain amygdala control so-called primitive or emotional responses of the limbic system, and the sense of smell.

The link may be no more than a matter of visual similarity, but wouldn't it be interesting if science found that almonds had the potential to influence lower brain function? Herbalists at various times have made such a link.

Hildegard of Bingen, writing in the twelfth century, states that almond fruits 'fill the brain'. Contemporary American herbalist Matthew Wood quotes Dr Fernie (1914): 'Persons who can readily digest these products [almonds] are believed to derive from them a quickening of the intellect in its magnetism, and in keenness, or argumentative force.'

Use almonds for...

Bought almonds come in a number of styles – whole, with or without skin, in halves, as flakes, ground, as an essence and as the oil. Roasted, salted and sugared forms are available to buy or can readily be made at home.

For medicinal use we prefer to start with the raw whole nut. Almonds become much easier to digest (and tastier) if you soak them in water overnight before eating. Some people find the skins irritating in the throat and digestive tract, in which case rub the skins off the soaked almonds or blanch by dropping them in boiling water for a few minutes.

Almond milk is gluten-free, dairy-free and almost carbohydrate-free. It is our favourite milk substitute and is an inexpensive home-made option for specialist diets, including for diabetes. It can be taken for constipation, inflammation of the intestines, including ulcerative colitis and irritable bowel, and for Crohn's disease.

Sweet almond oil is used in massage, and is a mild and gentle carrier for essential oils. It has high omega-3, and applied to dry skin is rejuvenating and toning (and much cheaper than asses' milk!).

Internally the oil is soothing and gently laxative (it is mild enough for children), and again is mollifying for intestinal spasm and moistens the respiratory system. It can be used for coughs and bronchial conditions, and was the old remedy for pleurisy, in which the lungs become dry.

To make marzipan (the medieval marchpane), dry the whole nuts and reduce them to a flour in a grinder or a pestle and mortar. Add a small amount of water to the flour to make your almond paste or add rose or orange water. Note that the milk or paste only last a day or two in the fridge.

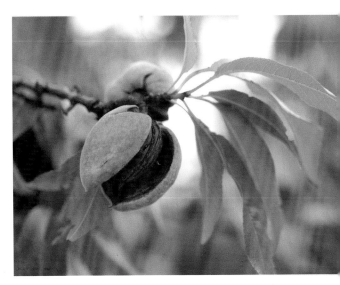

A comprehensive meta-analysis in 2016 found that 'The consumption of [almond] nuts as part of a healthy diet should be encouraged to help in the maintenance of healthy blood lipid levels and reduce the risk of heart disease.'

The oil newly pressed out of Sweet Almonds is a mitigator of pain and all manner of aches. ... The oil of Almonds makes smooth the hands and faces of delicate persons, and cleanseth the skin from all spots and pimples.
– Gerard (1597)

Almond milk

Soak 1 cup of **raw almonds** in water overnight. Pour off the soaking water and rinse the almonds well, then put them in a blender with 3 cups of filtered or spring **water**. Blend until smooth.

Pour through a fine strainer to remove the solids. The liquid is best used straightaway.

Options: Blend with a few dates if you like your milk with a hint of sweetness, or try adding a piece of vanilla bean. Alternatively the strained milk can be flavoured with a few drops of vanilla extract, rose water or orange blossom water. Almond milk is great for making hot cocoa drinks, milk shakes and puddings like blancmange.

The leftover almond granules can be eaten, or mixed with a little rosewater or vinegar and used as a face scrub and exfoliator.

Almond milk
• dairy substitute
• constipation
• ulcerative colitis
• irritable bowel
• dry cough

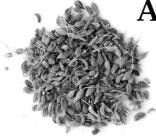

Aniseed, anise *Pimpinella anisum*

Like its botanical cousins fennel and dill, anise earns its keep in the medicine chest as well as the spice rack. It freshens the breath, aids digestion, and can be used to treat coughs. It also has a strong reputation as an aphrodisiac.

Apiaceae (Umbelliferae) Carrot family

Description: Annual plant with flat leaves, growing up to 1m (3ft) tall. Umbels of small white flowers are followed by aromatic brownish fruits.

Distribution: Native to western Asia; mainly grown in India and the Mediterranean.

Related species: Many plants in this family are used for food and medicine. Fennel (*Foeniculum vulgare*) is the most similar in flavour to aniseed. Star anise (*Illicium verum*) is not related but has a similar flavour.

Parts used: Seeds, botanically called fruit.

Anise seeds makes the breath modest and pleasant to the taste. ... dispels flatulence from the belly. ... it brings milk to the women and increases their desire for unchasteness. These seeds make appetite for eating and still belching.
– Fuchs (1543)

Aniseed needs a hot, long summer to ripen, making it difficult to bring to fruition in Britain, though it was well known in the boiled sweet, aniseed balls (which are now made with a synthetic). The leading commercial use of aniseed today is as a sweet flavouring for alcoholic drinks such as absinthe, anisette, pastis, ouzo and arak.

You may use aniseed at home to add a characteristic light liquorice flavour to cakes. If you do, you are following in old footsteps. The Roman natural historian Pliny the Elder (AD 23–79) wrote: 'Be it green or dried it [anise] is wanted for all conserves and flavourings.'

A simple grain and lard cake laced with aniseed and other spices was the Roman *mustaceae*, which was eaten as a cleanser after heavy, rich meals, especially at weddings. Mrs Grieve mentions the claim that *mustaceae* is the origin of modern spiced wedding cakes.

Use aniseed for...

Using anise as a breath freshener or digestive after eating is probably as old as the plant's origins in ancient Egypt or India. The first original herbal written in English, William Turner's *Herbal* of 1551, says: 'Anyse maketh the breth sweter and swageth payne.'

Aniseed works on the digestive system as a whole, not just the breath. It had a reputation in classical Roman times as *Solamen intestinorum*, or soother of the stomach. Anise reduces intestinal spasm, including hiccups, eases indigestion and bloating and also loosens phlegm. Commission E, the expert panel that advises the German government on herbs, endorses anise as an expectorant and cough suppressant.

Anise cuts bronchial secretions and has a reputation for treating asthma. Herbalist Matthew Wood suggests it for 'hard, dry, painful spasmodic coughs with phlegm sticking' (John Gerard called this 'the old cough').

As a weak tea it is safe for babies and young children, for colic or breathing problems. Otherwise, the seeds are chewed, or made into a tincture, fomentation or poultice. In 1597 Gerard summarised then-current thinking on aniseed:

The seed wasteth and consumeth winde, and is good against belchings and upbraidings of the stomacke, alaeith gripings of the belly, provoketh urine gently, maketh abundance of milke, and stirreth up bodily lust.

Gerard's last few words are supported by modern research. Aniseed (and star anise) is known to be rich in anethole, which has similar actions to the female sex hormone oestrogen. Anise indeed increases milk flow and assists in delivery, soothes menstrual cramps and stimulates libido.

Anise has a reputation as an aphrodisiac in Sanskrit as well as classical Greek and Roman texts. Perhaps the English word 'appetite' hints at more than an increased desire for food?

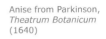

Anise from Parkinson, *Theatrum Botanicum* (1640)

Aniseed has gained a slightly dangerous reputation through its use to give a sweet flavour to absinthe, the death-or-glory drink of many French Impressionist artists. However, it is thujone from the wormwood in absinthe that was addictive and dangerous, not the aniseed.

Some Annis-seed be sweete, and some more bitter,/ For pleasure these, for medicine those are fitter.
– Harington (1607)

Like fennel, aniseed is a spice with a built-in feel-good factor. It helps us overcome the stresses of illness, so that more energy can be directed towards healing.
– Hedley & Shaw (1996)

Three spice powder
Mix equal parts of powdered **aniseed**, **ginger** and **black pepper**. **Dose:** half a teaspoonful mixed with a little local **honey** to make a paste. If you are diabetic or want to avoid honey for any reason, simply stir half a teaspoon of the powder into hot water as a drink.

Aniseed and thyme tea
Use ½ teaspoonful each of **aniseed** and **thyme** in a cup of hot water; cover and brew for 5 minutes, then strain and add a teaspoonful of honey. Slowly sip 2 tablespoonsful every half hour or hour. This gentle remedy is especially good for infants and young children.

Aniseed snaps
Heat 1 cup **molasses or golden syrup** to boiling point. Pour it over half a cup of **butter**, and stir until melted. Sift and stir in: 3¼ cups of **flour**, ½ teaspoon **bicarbonate of soda**, 1 tablespoon **aniseed powder** and 1 teaspoon **salt**. Roll out as thinly as possible, in small batches and cut out with a biscuit cutter. Bake at 190° for 8 to 10 minutes. For a spicier biscuit, use three spice powder (above) instead of just aniseed.

Three spice powder
• hayfever
• allergic rhinitis
• weak digestion
• head colds

Aniseed & thyme tea
• colds
• coughs
• breathing difficulties
• colic
• weak digestion

Aniseed snaps
• weak digestion
• poor appetite

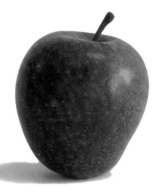

Apple *Malus communis, M. domestica*

Apples are among the most digestible of natural foods, with the ability to satisfy both hunger and thirst, settle the digestion and soothe the gastrointestinal tract. They are also somewhat astringent (crab apples very much so), making them anti-diarrhoeal, while their pectin has valuable cholesterol-reducing effects and their flavonoids are claimed to reduce risks in some cancers.

Rosaceae
Rose family

Description: A small deciduous tree, 3–10m (10–30ft) tall, with spring blossoms of tender white and pink, followed by autumn fruits, with creamy white flesh and up to 15 seeds or pips.

Distribution: Native to West Asia, and now thought to originate in the Caspian and Kazakhstan. Widely grown commercially in temperate areas with coldish winters and long summers.

Related species: Crab apple (*Malus sylvestris, Pyrus malus*) is a north European native ('crab' is an Old Norse term for scrub) and is a bracing forerunner of many eating apples.

Parts used: Fruit.

Does an apple a day really keep the doctor away?

The first expression of the idea in England is more recent than you might think, from 1866. The phrase recorded was 'Eat an apple on going to bed. And you'll keep the doctor from earning his bread.' A bit unzippy compared to the proverb we now use, but eating apples before sleep was a Victorian tradition, especially in the West Country, where apple dumplings were regular evening fare.

We will look at the reasons why apples are indeed wonderful for domestic medicine, but before that let us take a quick trip across the Atlantic for some context.

In an excellent essay on apples in his book *The Botany of Desire* (2002), Michael Pollan reminds us that in America until Prohibition apples were for drinking rather than eating. Every rural farmstead had its own orchard and cider press (much the same was true then in England). Cider gave sweetness when sugar was hard to come by, was easy to make at home, and yielded an appetising and of course intoxicating drink. Tea and coffee were scarce, and water was unsafe by comparison.

By the end of the nineteenth century the successful cloning of apple varieties like Jonathan and Delicious, along with the ability to transport apples by rail across the country and to refrigerate them, altered the rules of the game.

Temperance was gaining support, and the apple industry decided to change tack: apples were now for eating! And the slogan the public relations people came up with was 'an apple a day…' Today the average American consumes about 44lb (20kg) of apples a year, fresh or in foods and drinks.

So it's all about a successful PR campaign? Only partly, as apples have a much longer therapeutic past than this.

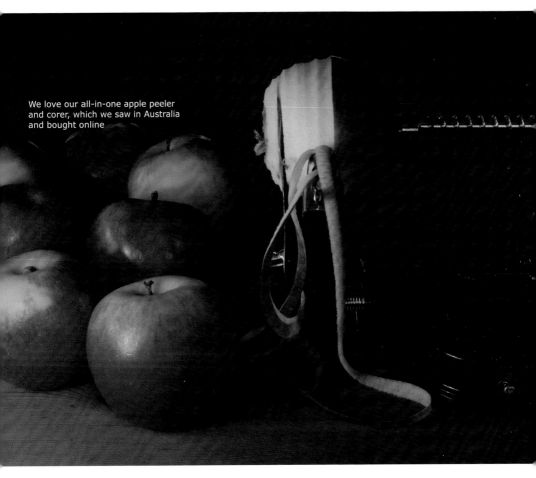

We love our all-in-one apple peeler and corer, which we saw in Australia and bought online

Apples proliferate in a huge number of varieties (over 7,000 in some estimates), not to mention wild native forms like the English crab apple (*Malus sylvestris, Pyrus malus*). Some apples are sweet, some tart; some are for cooking, some for the table; some make cider, vinegar or spirits.

All have a wealth of pectins, fructose, amino acids, vitamins and minerals, low calories (about 80 calories per apple), little fat and a good amount of pectin fibre. Moreover, apple is one of the most easily digestible natural foods: the naturopath Dr Fernie, in 1895, estimated that its complete digestion took only 85 minutes. Mrs Grieve (1931) agreed, and added that the sugar of a sweet apple is 'practically a pre-digested food' as it enters the bloodstream.

Another feature of apple is that the acids (malic and tartaric), once in the stomach form alkalines that cool the digestion and serve to limit the appetite. This is why apples make such good and satisfying snacks, while as

I am glad the new cook begins so well. Good Apple Pies are a considerable part of our domestic happiness.
– Jane Austen (1815)

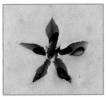

A cut apple shows the signature five-pointed star of the Rose family

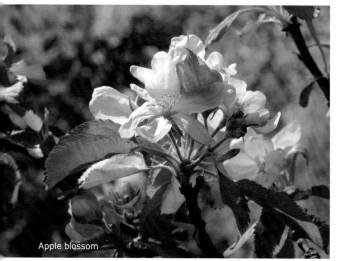

Apple blossom

a cooked sauce also counter rich meat tastes. Hence the apple put in the roast pig's mouth, perhaps.

Use apples for…

In terms of its digestive benefits, apple is 'amphoteric', meaning that it balances extremes, whether of constipation or diarrhoea. Folk wisdom is that cooked apple works for constipation but raw, grated apple is best for diarrhoea – indeed, perhaps the best simple remedy for infantile diarrhoea.

If you don't have your own trees, try to buy organic apples. Non-organic are heavily treated with pesticides, insecticides and so on. These accumulate on the apple skin and just beneath, and are locked in by waxing the surface (especially in North America).

As children are taught, eating the skin is good for you because the 'goodness' is concentrated there, but the proviso is that the skin is uncontaminated. Washing or rubbing the skin of non-organic apples may not be enough to render them chemical-free.

The other proviso is that you or your children chew the apple well, so that effective digestion begins in the mouth. This is good exercise for the jaw and benefits the teeth, as acids in apple help loosen plaque. Should we add dentists to doctors in apple-a-day formulas?

The world's healthiest breakfast is sometimes said to be muesli with fresh fruit. The Bircher-Benner clinic in Zurich long ago settled on a muesli with whole, flaked cereals soaked in water overnight, and raw grated and unskinned apple, prepared on the spot.

Apple is unusually versatile, being satisfying as both food and drink; it is tasty and nutritious whether raw or cooked, baked, stewed or boiled, in a pie, a fruit salad, a jelly, a strudel, a butter, a compote, a fool or a chutney. The juice is healthy by itself and as a cider and a vinegar; it is also distilled into the spirits calvados and applejack.

Apple is a satisfying thirst quencher, almost as effective as water (it is about 85% water by volume), and on a cellular level too. Apple juice is good to drink when there is hoarseness or coughs – in fact for almost any type of illness or indisposition.

In addition to balancing stomach activity, fibre in the pectin helps lower blood cholesterol levels, especially the potentially artery-clogging LDL. This means benefits for heart health and the circulation, while slower production of blood sugar is good news for those with diabetes and hypoglycaemia.

Proponents claim anti-cancer benefits from the antioxidant effects of apple, pointing to its high flavonoid content, especially of quercetin. Large-scale clinical research in the US has shown that eating apples did reduce risks for lung, colon and rectal cancers.

A word of caution here: from experience you will know that eating unripe apples leads to gut ache. And apple seeds, with their cyanide, are potentially poisonous. But relax, you'd need to take kilos' worth to be in trouble, and heating effectively disables the poison. Externally, a poultice of raw, grated apple can be applied to painful or swollen eyes; a poultice of cooked apple is equally good on bodily aches and pains.

In ancient Rome, apples and cloves went into a beauty treatment, prepared with lanolin. This goo or unguent was applied to the skin, literally as a 'pomade'. Bruised, browned apples were a form of antiseptic used in British folk medicine, and were applied to styes or chilblains even in the mid-twentieth century.

And if you tire of the apple-a-day theme, how about Prince Ahmed's apple? In the *Arabian Nights* story, the Prince buys a magical apple in Samarkhand that is a cure for every ill. It may be significant that this fabled city was close by the source of the original wild apples of Kazakhstan.

I frequently pluck wild apples of so rich and spicy a flavor that I wonder all orchardists do not get a scion from that tree, and I fail not to bring home my pockets full.
– Thoreau (1862)

Nowadays … the wonderfully-rich gene pool of the apple is being dumbed down for commercial reasons … to the miserable exclusion of older, wiser, more subtle varieties which are gradually becoming extinct.
– Roberts (2001)

Grated apple and ginger

Grate 2 **apples** coarsely (with the peel on), then finely grate about a teaspoonful of **fresh root ginger**. Mix together in a bowl and eat straightaway to settle an upset stomach or when recovering from illness. Particularly good after a bout of vomiting and diarrhoea.

Spicy apple sauce

Wash **apples** and cut into quarters. Put into a saucepan with just enough **water** to keep them from burning, and cook over low to moderate heat until the apples are soft and mushy. Put through a coarse strainer to remove the pips, etc.

Add a spoonful of **cinnamon powder**, a pinch of **allspice**, a sprinkle of **salt**, and **brown sugar** to taste. Some people like to add lemon juice and a bit of butter. If you are a cold person or the weather is cold, eat the apple sauce hot.

Grated apple & ginger
• upset stomach
• convalescence
• diarrhoea
• inflammation
• nausea

Spicy apple sauce
• upset stomach
• convalescence
• weak digestion
• constipation

Arrowroot *Maranta arundinacea* **Maranta, Obedience plant**

Marantaceae
Maranta family

Description: A perennial herbaceous plant native to the Caribbean and adjacent mainland South America, which grows to 2m (6ft).

Other arrowroots: Queensland, African or purple arrowroot (*Canna edulis* [Canna]); East Indian arrowroot (*Curcuma angustifolia* [Zingiber]); Brazilian arrowroot (*Manihot esculenta* [Cassava, manioc]); Japanese arrowroot, kudzu (*Pueraria lobata*); Indian, South Sea, Polynesian, Tahiti or Hawaian arrowroots (*Tacca leontopetaloides* [Tacca]); Florida or wild arrowroot, coontie palm (*Zamia floridana*).

Parts used: Tubers.

The real reason the British love arrowroot is to support their colonies.
– attributed to Napoleon Bonaparte

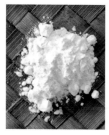

In our kitchens we store tropical fire in the form of powdered ginger and chilli, but there is also a category of tropical bland, well exemplified in arrowroot. More neglected now than by our Victorian forebears, arrowroot is still useful for making quick sauces and jellies, and medicinally can soothe the heat of an upset stomach, diarrhoea or irritated skin.

Arrowroot has thin, reed-like stems (*arundinacea* in the Latin name means 'reedy'), paddle-shaped leaves and small white flowers, but the main feature of interest is its fleshy cylindrical tubers, mistakenly called roots.

The English 'arrowroot' comes from the Aruwak Indians of the pre-colonial West Indies, who valued these tubers as a starch-rich food and made poultices with them for poison arrow wounds.

The 'true arrowroot' is Maranta, but many tubers grown around the tropics and subtropics also known as arrowroot belong in other botanical families (see left). Adulteration of arrowroot, often by the cheaper cassava or potato starch, has always been and is still a commercial problem.

The tubers are harvested after a year, then are washed, peeled, soaked, crushed and dried in the sun. This process yields a fine white powder, with 25% or more starch content, very little protein and some fibre.

The Victorians were the true believers in arrowroot as a food for convalescents, infants and those who could not hold down anything other than a bland sauce or thin soup. The arrowroot habit persisted: our copy of the *Kenya Settlers' Cookery Book* (12th edition, 1957) has recipes for arrowroot cream, custard and gruel.

Its botanically simple molecular structure means arrowroot has a lower boiling point than the more complex corn or wheat starch, and readily forms a jelly with modest heating. Because it lacks proteins it also stays clear when cooked.

Today, we'd claim arrowroot as a low-salt, protein- and gluten-free starch, which can meet the needs of people with a wheat allergy.

Use arrowroot for...
Arrowroot is a demulcent, and its mucilage coats inflamed internal passageways of the mouth and digestive system, thus protecting them. It is readily digested and sits easily in the stomach, hence the fame of arrowroot soups, gruels

and jellies. Its alkalinity helps to harmonise an over-acid stomach, and it is a useful home remedy for colic and diarrhoea.

Externally, apply the powder to irritated skin or to rashes. While it does not heal bites or wounds (or poisons), having little antiseptic value in itself, as a fine powder it will absorb any moisture and reduce friction. It helps athlete's foot by keeping your feet dry, and is soothing for heat rash.

Arrowroot powder makes a good dry shampoo – simply massage a little into the hair, then comb or brush out.

Note that some people are allergic to arrowroot on the skin, and it may exacerbate the conditions it usually improves. Try a little at first. If in doubt, and if rashes get worse, stop using it.

We'd argue arrowroot deserves a better fate than being known as making probably the driest and most boring biscuit in the world.

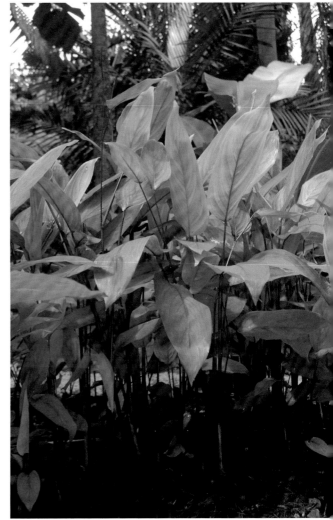

Arrowroot growing in Singapore

Arrowroot pudding

Put 250ml **almond milk** (or regular milk) in a saucepan. Take enough out to make a thin paste with 1 tablespoon **arrowroot powder** and ½ teaspoon **vanilla extract**, then heat the rest, bringing to the boil. Add 1 to 2 tablespoons **brown sugar**, ½ teaspoonful **butter or coconut oil**, then pour onto the arrowroot mixture. Stir until smooth and thickening up, then pour into a bowl. Can be eaten warm, or chilled.

Arrowroot powder

Arrowroot powder can be used as is as a foot and body powder. You can also brush it through hair as a dry shampoo. If you want to add fragrance, stir in a few drops of essential oil and sieve; store in a jar.

Arrowroot pudding
- gut inflammation
- weak digestion
- diarrhoea
- convalescence

Arrowroot powder
- heat rash
- fungal infections
- dry shampoo

Banana *Musa* x *paradisiaca* and other spp.

Musaceae
Banana family

Description: Tender evergreen perennial herb, with large palm-like leaves, and growing to 2–6m high (6.5–20ft); hanging, red 'cigar' flower and bunches of 'finger' fruit that are green on the branch and yellow on ripening.

Distribution: Probably originating in India and SE Asia, now cultivated widely in the tropics and subtropics; 40 wild species and over 300 cultivars are known. Dessert bananas are descended from the wild species *Musa acuminata*, while the plantains and other cooking bananas also have genes from *M. balbisiana*.

Parts used: Fruit, skin (leaves and root have various applications in banana-growing areas).

Found in kitchens around the world, bananas are the most popular fruit and the largest, most productive herb of all. They are a good source of potassium, and a mood food. The skins are also useful for treating insect bites and age spots.

Banana is not really a tree but the largest herb known – a perennial with a 'trunk' of overlapping and semi-rigid coarse leaves. It is the most productive herb too, with 10 to 20 bananas per hand, up to 15 hands per bunch, and several bunches per plant per year.

It is now the most popular fruit in the world. A survey showed that 95% of Britons buy bananas regularly, and over thirty years ago it supplanted the apple as the nation's favourite fruit. Britons, like Americans, eat on average two to three bananas a week.

Global exports of bananas reached 118 million tons in 2017, up from

68mt in 2000, although it should be added that most bananas grown are not traded at all, being subsistence food for small farmers in the tropics and subtropics.

Use bananas for…
Why are bananas so popular? It is partly the convenience of the wonderful natural packaging, and the fact you can eat the whole contents – there are no seeds (all bananas are grown from suckers, so are genetically clones of the parent plant; seeds are vestigial).

Bananas are rightly acknowledged as a superb source of instant, absorbable energy in the form of glucose, fructose and sucrose – excellent for athletes and children. Reputedly they are richer in minerals than any other soft fruit except strawberries, almost as high in pectin fibre as apples, and have a good complement of vitamins.

Bananas are now known to have bioavailable tryptophan, an amino acid the brain uses to make serotonin. Serotonin is a neurotransmitter that controls gut movements and also affects mood, appetite, learning and the memory.

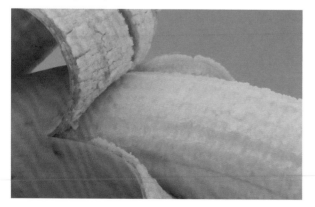

Bananas are a cooling food, and effective at settling the stomach in most people. Banana purée is a safe infant food, and banana smoothies with honey are touted as a hangover cure.

As a ready source of potassium, bananas are useful in osteroporosis diets, as restoration of potassium levels implies less loss of calcium. This potassium effect is also seen in lower blood pressure, stress and hypoglycaemia, through reduction of the damaging LDL cholesterol in the blood and raising that of the beneficial HDL.

Bananas may be used to help treat anaemia as their iron content stimulates production of haemoglobin in the blood.

Finally, don't just discard your banana skin. Its inside is cooling on a bruise or sunburn, and for mosquito bites, as an emergency poultice or for treating liver spots. But, sorry, those 1960s stories about the skins' hallucinogenic properties were just a pipe dream.

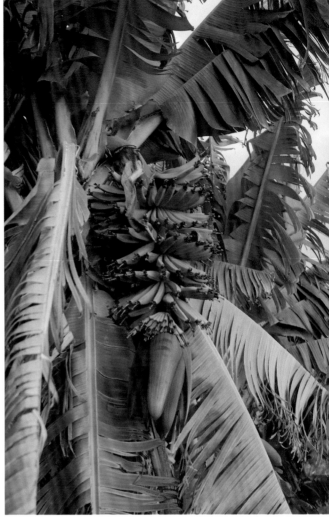

Bananas growing in Madeira, February

Banana almond smoothie
Blend until smooth: 1 ripe **banana**, 1½ cups of **almond milk** and ¼ teaspoonful of **cardamom powder.**

Options: Add a teaspoon of **vanilla extract** to increase the feel-good factor, or a teaspoonful of **honey** if you want it sweeter.

Banana skin
Peel a banana and rub the inside of the **skin** on insect bites, sunburn or any hot itchy skin condition for cooling relief. Banana skins can also be used daily on the backs of the hands to lighten age and liver spots.

Banana almond smoothie
• low mood
• low energy
• hypoglycaemia
• muscle cramps

Banana skin
• insect bites
• sunburn
• age spots
• liver spots

Barley *Hordeum distichon, H. vulgare*

Graminae (Poaceae)
Grass family

Description: Annual grain, to about 1m (3ft) tall, with hollow stem, spear-shaped leaves, ears bearing twin rows of seeds and long awns or bristles; flexible (cf. wheat), and when blown in the wind resembles 'a sea of grass'.

Distribution: Once a wild plant in the Middle East, now widespread in temperate areas worldwide, including at altitude (eg Tibet); arrived in East before wheat.

Related species: Six-rowed barley (*H. vulgare*) is used in Chinese medicine; various wild species, eg wall barley (*H. murinum*).

Parts used: Seed in various forms.

A traditional approach from Britain for soothing the urinary tract is barley water. This has been used in much the same way that cranberry juice has in North America. They work in different ways but achieve similar results. Barley water may be used in all cases where frequency, dysuria, or another distressing symptom occurs.
– Hoffmann (2003)

Barley is an ancient grain, used for at least 10,000 years, and a universal staple for bread, beer, porridge and broths; barley water has probably been used medicinally for just as long. In various forms, barley is beneficial both for the weak, as in babies or convalescents, and for the strong, as in today's tennis stars and yesterday's gladiators. Its benefits include soothing the throat, stomach, intestinal and urinary tracts, and reducing inflammations and swellings, diarrhoea and constipation.

Barley has been gathered, grown and used for ten millennia, longer than wheat, rice or rye, mankind's other major temperate cereals. As such an old staple, barley's uses inevitably encompassed both food and medicine, and it contributes to bread, beer, porridge and broths, barley water and malt.

Some of the domestic medicinal uses of barley are well worth reviving, and that forgotten bag or box of barley grains, pearl barley or flakes in your kitchen cupboard deserves another look.

Barley is sold in various styles, including whole grain, flour (patent barley), pearl (with most of the outer layers removed until the shiny white endosperm remains), flake, grit and other forms (see p21 for details). Barley sugar, however, has long since ceased to have any connection with the cereal.

One interesting thing about barley is that it works both for the very fit and the very weak. The link of barley water and Wimbledon is well known (see p20), but possibly less familiar is that Roman gladiators consumed barley products in training for the arena.

The gladiator diet was basically vegetarian, with high proteins and carbohydrates. One group of gladiators became the 'hordearii', or 'barley eaters', after *hordeum*, the official name for barley. The famous physician Galen was the doctor in Rome's gladiator school.

In Egypt the Pyramids were built by slave labour subsisting on a diet of bread, beer and onions; two of these were derived from barley. Our term 'booze' may well come from the name for the barley-based beer of the Fellaheen.

Barley water remains a valuable first non-milk food for infants, helping in the breakdown of milk products and soothing the stomach; it is equally palatable for convalescents. Sometimes called Scottish or Jewish pencillin,

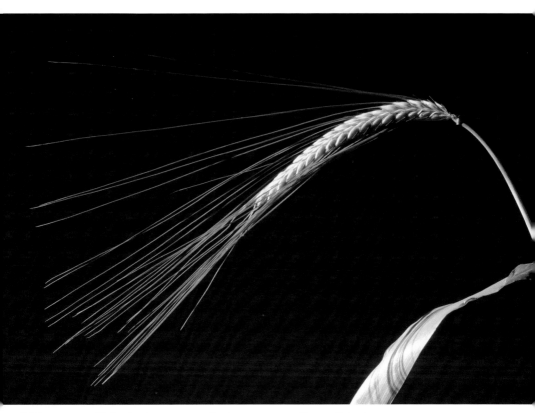

chicken soup with barley is a classic dish for nourishing the unwell.

In medieval Germany Hildegard of Bingen recommended bathing in barley water for recovering patients. Another external use for barley flour or paste is in the form of a poultice, applied to inflammations and swellings, when barley's cooling qualities are fully utilised.

The difference between making barley water to sip or bathe in and barley broth or porridge to eat is largely one of how much boiling is done: cooking breaks down the grains more and the mix becomes more viscous and soup-like, but the forms are equally medicinal. Sprouted barley grains can be grown into barley grass (which goes well with wheatgrass), high in chlorophyll, or the sprouts can be made into malt or malt extract through a process of germination, steeping, kilning and converting into a brewer's wort. The wort then can be brewed into beer or whisky, or be evaporated to leave a malt extract.

The Victorians were the champions of malt, with their malted milks, cakes, jellies and biscuits. The last century has not been kind to malt as a foodstuff, though malting barley is prized more than ever for making high-grade whisky, and malt vinegar.

And whoever is so sick that the whole body is weak should cook barley in rapidly boiling water, pour the water in a tub, and bathe in it. This the person should do often, until cured, and the tissue grows strong and healthy.
– Hildegard of Bingen (1098–1179)

[Barley water is a] *... most elegant, and grateful beverage, which is extremely useful in the gravel, stone, strangury, and heat of urine; likewise in fevers of the ardent kind, and other acute disorders where cooling and diluting are necessary.*
– Meyrick (1789)

Use barley for...

Along with good amounts of vitamins B and E, calcium, potassium, protein and starch, barley is a ready source of selenium, an antioxidant that protects against heart disease and is needed for normal growth.

In the form of barley water, barley is known as a supportive, gentle and alkaline treatment for urinary and kidney problems.

A friend of ours, diagnosed with urinary problems, cut out tea and coffee, and switched to fresh barley water, which he still takes to work with him in a vacuum flask every day. His problem was resolved long ago, and he finds he now enjoys the barley water for the taste and modest energy boost.

The effect of barley internally is also anti-inflammatory, anti-spasmodic and cooling, making it effective in cases of intestinal swellings or ulcers, irritable bowel, haemorrhoids and colitis. It eases the unpleasantness and distress of both constipation and diarrhoea, by relaxing the muscle of the stomach and intestinal lining.

Make barley water too for sore throats and add it to other herbs where a soothing action is recommended.

Barley supplies dietary fibre in the form of beta glucans, which has been shown to lower the 'bad' blood cholesterol LDL and thus improve some heart conditions. Barley has responded well in trials for hepatitis and type-2 diabetes.

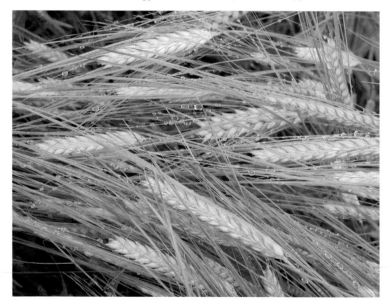

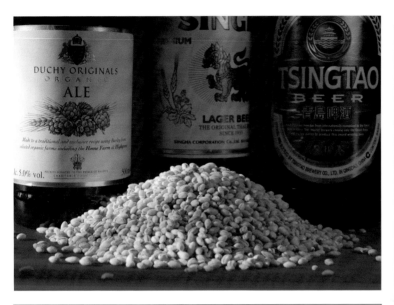

Barley in the kitchen
• Whole or hulled barley (for soups and stews) has some or all the bran removed
• Unground grain (Scotch barley)
• Pot barley has some bran removed
• Pearl barley is ground to whiteness (hence the name)
• Patent barley is meal from pearl barley, used as a thickener and to make infants' cereal foods
• Barley water was made at home by boiling pearl barley in water, cooled and sweetened; sometimes flavoured with orange or lemon (hence lemon barley water)
• Barley flakes, grits or nibs

Barley water

Put in a large saucepan: ½ cup **pot barley**, 5 cups **water,** a small piece of **cinnamon** stick and 1 or 2 teaspoons **grated ginger.**

Simmer for 20 minutes then cool and strain. Add the **juice of a lemon**, freshly squeezed.

Store in the fridge (keep for up to two days only), and drink 2 or 3 cups a day at room temperature. Extra lemon juice can be added just before drinking.

Barley soup

Put in a saucepan: 3 cups **water** and ½ cup **barley**. Simmer for half an hour.

Sauté 1 **onion** (finely diced), 1 teaspoon minced **garlic**, and ½ cup of sliced **mushrooms** until cooked, then add to the barley soup. Add **miso, tamari or sea salt** to taste. Add ½ cup chopped **parsley** and a handful of chopped **chives** or **spring onions**, cook for about a minute longer and then serve.

If someone is very weak and ill, strain the soup and just give them the broth.

Barley water
• kidney problems
• low energy
• urinary infections
• coughs
• convalescence
• haemorrhoids
• IBS

Barley soup
• convalescence
• blood sugar imbalances
• IBS
• colitis
• weakened energy
• low immunity
• haemorrhoids
• high cholesterol

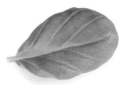

Basil *Ocimum basilicum, O. tenuiflorum* syn. *O. sanctum*

**Lamiaceae
(Labiatae)
Mint family**

In addition to its universal presence in pastas and pizzas, basil has old medicinal uses in treating head, stomach and lung disorders and fevers, and these may well be extended by recent research findings. Perhaps above all, basil lifts the spirits.

Description: Aromatic annual (*O. basilicum*), growing to about 50cm (20in) with shiny dark green leaves and groups of small white flowers; or tender perennial (*O. tenuiflorum*) growing to 1m (3ft).

Distribution: Probably native to India, now grown around the world commercially, in gardens and as a pot plant.

Basil species:
Sweet basil (*Ocimum basilicum*) also has a purple form. Holy basil or tulsi (*O. tenuiflorum*) was previously called *O. sanctum*. There are over 150 basil varieties, including tree or shrub basil (*Ocimum gratissimum*), with medicinal and insect-repellent uses; bush basil (*O. minimum*), African camphor basil (*O. kilimandscharicum*); lemon basil (*O. americanum*); Thai lemon basil (*O. citriodorum*) and Asian basil (*O. canum*).

Parts used: Leaves, flowers, essential oil.

There was a time just a few decades ago when *pesto* was only known as a basil and pine nut sauce made in the Genoa region, and *soupe au pistou* was a specialism of Nice. But the later twentieth century saw a universal declaration of love for pasta, pizza, salads and their essential components, tomato and basil.

Sweet basil is an annual aromatic herb that is on a peak of popularity as an ingredient of the most favoured fast foods of the day. This may be new, but its gastronomic virtues were well known to the ancient civilisations of the Mediterranean, Egypt, India and in China and the Far East.

Basil as a medicinal herb may have been overshadowed in the feeding frenzy, but it has a venerable history of benign use in the same geographical areas. We think it should be more widely known today, echoing the herbalist John Hill, writing in 1812: '… little used, but it deserves to be much more. A tea of the green plant is excellent against all obstructions. No simple is more effective for gently promoting the menses.'

In passing, we should confirm Hill's comment and note that as it encourages menstruation, basil in the form of a tea or essential oil should be avoided in pregnancy. Eating pizzas, though, is fine!

In India, probably where the plant originated, basil is a sacred herb, second only to the lotus. *Tulsi* or holy basil is dedicated to Vishnu and Krishna, and offers divine protection. It is a *rasayana*, meaning a plant that supports life and promotes health, by balancing the energies of the body and sustaining the life force.

Tulsi is grown in pots in most Hindu households, and is part of everyday ritual. It is favoured for drinks rather than in food, unlike sweet basil, and is not so pleasant to the taste. In India, as in southern Africa, basil in pots or burnt dried is also used to keep away flies and mosquitoes.

In Indian folk medicine, basil leaf tea is a home remedy for colds and bronchitis, and a tea made of the seeds is taken as a diuretic. A winter hot drink is *tulsi ki chah*, combining basil leaves, pounded ginger and honey. Basil leaf tea is also taken in India as an expectorant for removing mucus, and to calm an upset stomach.

If in India holy basil has an unassailable provenance, in Europe there has always been an ambivalence about sweet basil. On one hand, its name derives from the Greek *basilikon phuton*, denoting royal herb. This might, as one herbalist suggests, be because it was so useful a herb rather than an association with specific kings.

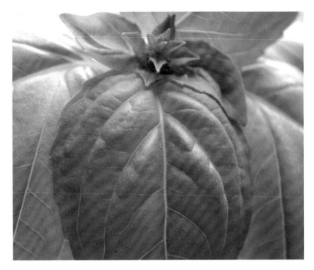

On the other hand, the name did resemble the less salubrious *basilicus*, the basilisk, a mythical reptile whose glance or breath meant instant death to its victims; in time the creature in question became a real one, the scorpion.

The conflation of the names had already begun in the time of classical writers like Theophrastus and Pliny, and, repeated for well over a millennium, became an entrenched belief. Medieval stories of basil causing scorpions to grow in the brain were accepted by 'rational' English herbalists like William Turner (1568).

But does basil's dual reputation as both useful and dangerous reflect merely an ancient linguistic confusion? Why was the contradiction worth sustaining?

One possibility might lie in the erotic and magical association of aromatic herbs, linking their warmth, scent and passion with deeper threats or suppressed sexual guilts. Basil itself was known for its sedative qualities in childbirth, and to promote production of milk and menses.

But perhaps a more reasoned account of the ambivalence towards basil can be made from its specific medicinal actions as both as stimulant and sedative for the nervous system.

Herbalist Matthew Wood notes that in the Mediterranean basil tea is used in the morning to energise the system and then in the evening to soothe it before sleep. He calls this an 'unusual and valuable fact'. Wood adds that basil can be either heating or cooling for influenza, a condition typified by intermittent swings to either extreme, as the body needs.

It is good for the stryking of a sea dragon, and the stynge of scorpiones. The sede dronken is good for them that brede melancholii; and for them that are puffed up with wind. ... The most part use Basil and eat it with oyle & [vine] gare, sauce for a fowl or chicken.
– Turner (1568)

The Physicall properties are, to procure a cheerefull and merry heart, whereunto the seed is chiefly used in pouder, &c. and is most used to that, and to no other purpose.
– Parkinson (1629)

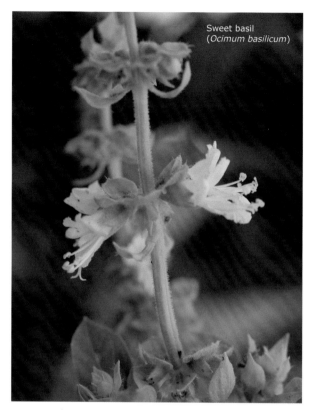

Sweet basil
(*Ocimum basilicum*)

Use basil for...

Beginning at the head, basil leaf tea is a pleasant treatment for a headache caused by nervous tension or indigestion. The smell is uplifting and the aromatic oils penetrate a head cold or fever.

John Gerard expressed the traditional positive view in 1597: 'The smell of Basill is good for the heart and for the head … it taketh away sorrowfulnesse, which cometh of melancholie, and maketh a man merrie and glad.' That is an excellent description of depression and a way to relieve it.

Another way to lighten headaches is to soak a cloth in basil tea and use it as a head compress. Stuffed noses were once treated in Europe by a basil snuff from crumbled dried leaves – the same remedy is found in southern Africa.

The juice of basil has an old use for earache, from the time of the classical Greek authors. The tea makes a good mouthwash for rinsing and gargling in cases of bleeding gums and mouth thrush.

David Winston describes how basil stimulates cerebral circulation and the memory. He notes that in Ayurveda it is a specific remedy for the 'mental fog' that accompanies chronic cannabis smoking. He favours basil with cerebral stimulants like rosemary and ginkgo for cloudy thinking in menopause, for poor memory, and ADD and ADHD.

The dried leaves are much used as an ingredient in cephalic, and herb-snuffs, and other sternutatory powders.
– Meyrick (1789)

It specifically increases prana and the life force. Its pungency and penetrating nature clears dampness and toxic ama that can cause chest infections and fevers. Its special power is to be used in all fevers regardless of their cause.
– Pole (2006)

Another contemporary herbalist, David Winston, gives basil a chapter in his book on *Adaptogens*, a category of multi-acting and even paradoxical herbs that intelligently lift depressed parts of the system or balance over-stimulated parts.

Our postmodern age is perhaps the first in which the positivity in apparent contradiction can be celebrated and a concept like 'adaptogens' make explanatory sense. Basil typifies the process.

It can also be taken to strengthen the stomachs of patients recovering from chemotherapy, and is now known as a radioprotective, ie protects against ionising radiation.

Basil helps clear mucus from the lungs and upper respiratory tract, and has a place in treatment of colic, irritable bowel and diarrhoea. Basil tea helps the body under a 'flu attack by encouraging sweating, thereby lowering the core temperature. In India basil is a fever herb *par excellence*.

Preliminary trials in the last two decades suggest new possibilities for basil in the treatment of type-2 diabetes and certain disorders of the immune system. Full-scale human clinical trials may yet confirm basil as a more diverse and sympathetic herb than traditionally thought, with its dangerous past perhaps becoming a bountiful future.

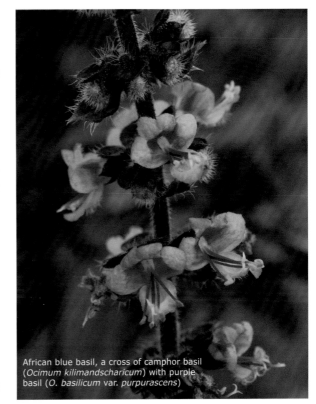
African blue basil, a cross of camphor basil (*Ocimum kilimandscharicum*) with purple basil (*O. basilicum* var. *purpurascens*)

Basil tea
Use a couple of sprigs of sweet, holy or other **basil** of your choice per mug of boiling water. Cover and steep for several minutes.

Basil pesto
This classic recipe is one of the tastiest ways to take basil. Traditionally ground by hand using a pestle, which gives the sauce its name.

Pound 2 cloves chopped **garlic** with 1 teaspoon **sea salt** to make a soft mush. Add 25g (1oz) lightly toasted **pine nuts**, then gradually add the leaves of a cupful of **sweet basil**, grinding until you have a silky paste. Stir in 50g (2oz) grated **Pecorino or Parmesan cheese** and 100ml (3½ fl oz) **extra virgin olive oil**. If you are making it in a blender or food processer, you will need to add more olive oil or other liquid. Use as a pasta sauce or serve over rice or vegetables.

Basil tea
- lifts the spirits
- headaches
- indigestion
- poor memory
- lack of concentration
- mild depression
- imbalances
- exposure to radiation

Basil pesto
- lifts the spirits
- poor memory
- lack of concentration
- mild depression
- exposure to radiation

Beetroot, red beet

Beta vulgaris, subsp. *vulgaris* convar. *vulgaris* var. *vulgaris*

**Amaranthaceae
Amaranth family**

Description:
Perennial, up to 1m
or even 1.5m (3–5ft)
high, with large and
dark red-veined green
leaves, enlarged red
bulbous root, and red
and greenish flowers.

Distribution: The
ancestral plant, Sea
beet (*Beta vulgaris*
subsp. *maritima*),
is found wild above
high-tide mark on
beaches in Europe,
parts of Middle East, to
India; other beets are
cultivated worldwide in
temperate zones.

Related species:
Leaf beets, *B. vulgaris*
subsp. *vulgaris* convar.
cicla (including spinach,
var. *cicla*; chard, var.
flaviscens); tuberous
beets, *B. vulgaris*,
subsp. *vulgaris* convar.
vulgaris (including
mangelwurzel, var.
crassa; sugar beet,
var. *altissima*).

Parts used: Root, leaf.

Beetroot or red beet is one of several successful cultivars of wild sea beet. A well-known salad or soup ingredient (as in borscht), it also has a medicinal history, including immune support and for anaemia, but also some controversial modern applications.

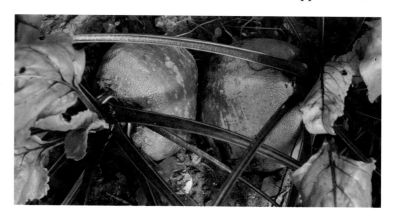

Wild sea beet was probably domesticated in Egypt in the second millennium BC, at much the same time as cabbage, carrots and asparagus. What has made beet so successful as a cultivated species is its adaptability and the readiness with which it offered cultivars. While spinach and chard originated in beet leaves, beetroot, sugar beet and mangelwurzels were bred out of beet tap roots.

Beetroot itself first emerged in imperial Roman times from selective breeding of red wild beet. It was known later as Roman beet, but only became a food in England in the seventeenth century.

John Gerard, in 1597, liked the leaves: 'The greater red Beete or Roman Beet, boyled and eaten with oyle, vinegre and pepper, is a most excellent and delicat sallad' – but he wasn't sure about the root: 'what might be made of the red and beautifull roote … I referre unto the curious and cunning cooke.'

In 1812, herbalist John Hill preferred the white beet for home medicinal use, red beet in his estimation being similar but less strong. Hill wrote that the 'juice of fresh beet-root is an excellent remedy for the head-ach, and tooth-ach when the whole jaw is affected; it is to be snuffed up the nose to promote sneezing'.

Hill's last remedy was repeating unchanged one from Dioscorides in first-century AD Greece. Greeks of that time also knew beet as a fever remedy, while in Rome at a similar period beetroot juice was used to treat dandruff and chilblains, as a wound dressing and for snake bite.

Use beetroot for…
Medicinally, eaten raw in a salad or lightly cooked, beet leaves are a liver cleanser. They contain lutein, which helps prevent macular degeneration, the leading cause of blindness in older adults, but also oxalic acid, which taken in excess inhibits calcium metabolism and can contribute to kidney stones.

If you find you have red urine after eating the root, don't worry: it is an indication that you have low stomach acid (see also vinegar, p181). The red derives from betanin, an anthocyanin similar to the red principle in wine; it has been found to assist the lymphatic system and be immune-supporting. White beet contains the similar betaine, which is a cleanser for the blood, liver and gallbladder. Beetroot has plentiful vitamins A, B-complex and C, and minerals, including iron and zinc.

Evidence is accumulating that taking high amounts of beetroot juice (measured in terms of glasses full rather than spoons) strengthens the body in cancer-treatment programmes, alongside other remedial treatment. On the other hand, beetroot as a government-recommended 'cure' for AIDS proved highly controversial – and unsuccessful – in South Africa in recent years.

A 2018 meta-study showed that regular intake of beetroot juice improved intermittent high-intensity exercise efforts by delaying depletion of phosphocreatine. Sports drink: a new use for the versatile beet?

… fantastic change, from the wild species in the sand to scarlet slices in vinegar.
– Grigson (1955)

As an easily digested food beetroots are ideal for those with sensitive stomachs, while their generally cooling and immune-stimulant actions also make them a useful addition to the menu for those suffering from colds, coughs and catarrh.
– Ody (2002)

Beetroot stains?
These are inevitable when handling the root, so try these household tips: apply lemon juice to red fingers before washing them with soap and hot water; beetroot stains on fabric can be rubbed with a slice of uncooked pear before washing; use diluted bleach on reddened cutting boards or containers.

Beetroot juice
Beetroot juice on its own is very strong, so try this combination. Juice a raw **beetroot,** with 2 **apples**, a stick of **celery** and a **carrot**. The proportions can be adjusted to taste. Drink a glass daily.

Borscht
Boil 1½ litres (3pts) of **water** or vegetable stock with a couple of **allspice**, a couple of **bay leaves** and 10 **black peppercorns** for 15 minutes, then remove the spices. Grate 4 red **beetroot**, a **carrot**, an **onion**, a **parsnip** and a **potato**. Add to the stock and simmer for 30 minutes or until the vegetables are soft. Blend until smooth and add a glass of **red wine** or a tablespoon of **red wine vinegar**. Serve with a dollop of **sour cream**.

Beetroot juice
• anaemia
• detoxifying
• immune support

Borscht
• anaemia

Bicarbonate of soda, baking soda

Bicarbonate of soda (baking soda) is universally known and used as a leavening (raising) agent in baking, but it also has many uses in household cleaning. In kitchen medicine its value is as an alkaliser and producer of carbon dioxide, offering ready help for domestic tummy upsets, stings and burns, for relieving gout and as a simple and inexpensive deodorant. A recent use is as a performance enhancer in explosive sports.

Description:
Bicarbonate of soda is sodium bicarbonate, a chemical compound with the formula $NaHCO_3$. It is a crystalline white solid but is usually kept as a fine powder. It is also known as sodium acid carbonate or sodium hydrogen carbonate.

Source: Sodium bicarbonate occurs naturally as nahcolite in association with volcanic activity.

Commercial production includes the mining of nahcolite, sourcing from trona and other minerals or isolation from naturally occurring brines such as natron. China is the largest producer, followed by the USA.

Never, under any circumstances, unless you wish entirely to destroy all flavour, and reduce your peas to pulp, boil them with soda. This favourite atrocity of the English kitchen cannot be too strongly condemned.
– Tabitha Tickletooth (1860)

The name bicarbonate of soda, bicarb or bread soda is used in many English-speaking countries, while baking soda is the North American term. Both differ from baking powder, which is bicarb plus an acidifying and a drying agent: see the panel on p30 for more detail.

Bicarb (as we will call it) is a naturally occurring mineral but also an alkali produced in the body by the pancreas, to neutralise acidic stomach secretions as they enter the small intestine.

In the kitchen, bicarb is mainly used as a leavening agent, as in soda bread, biscuits and cakes. It was combined with vinegar in Second World War eggless cake recipes, and is a necessary component of baking powder.

It also enlivens chlorophyll, making 'greens' like the brassicas much greener during cooking. Matthew remembers his Grandma Hale in the 1950s, boiling cabbage for an hour until mushy, then adding a pinch of bicarb to make it green again. No one told her she was destroying the vitamin B1 and C. She, like English cooks of the time, should have heeded Tabitha from a century before (see left).

Bicarb has many household uses besides cooking. Almost every American fridge contains an open box of baking soda to absorb the odours. Its gentle abrasion lends it to a variety of cleaning purposes, while its available alkalinity makes it useful in swimming pools to counteract chlorine.

Commercially, bicarb has wide application, including in medicine. It is prescribed for treating metabolic acidosis and gastric hyperacidity, as an alkalising agent for urine, for high potassium levels in the blood, and in some cases of poisoning and for overdose of certain drugs, including tricyclic antidepressants and aspirin. It is sometimes given intravenously for cardiac arrest.

Use bicarb for...

A familiar home medicinal use of bicarb is to settle the stomach acids after a big meal. It is generally safe to take (though it is unpleasant to the taste), but be aware that a small, burpy 'fizz' can become an internal explosion in some very rare cases.

Julie's parents knew an executive at the *National Geographic* in Washington DC who suffered a stomach rupture soon after taking baking soda in water for indigestion after a late meal. The victim underwent emergency surgery. After recovering he sued Church & Dwight, makers of the Arm & Hammer brand of baking soda, for insufficient warning on their labelling.

The manufacturer's defence in court was that millions of people had taken bicarb for tummy complaints for centuries, and this case was unique. A distended stomach could not expand any more when carbon dioxide was explosively released as the bicarb hit the victim's stomach acids.

Many of the age-old remedies and applications of bicarbonate of soda can be traced back ... to the knowledge possessed by the Ancient Egyptians.
– Briggs (2007)

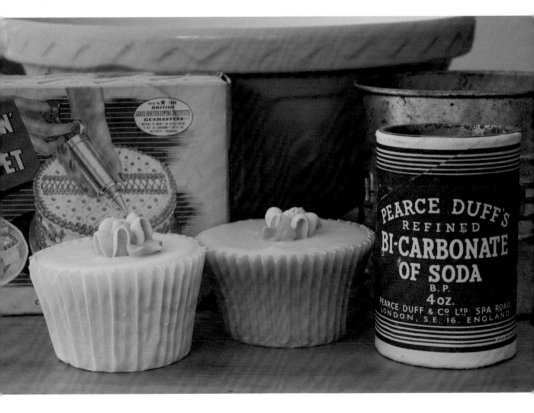

An excellent, practical use for sodium bicarbonate is its cleansing properties [for refrigerators]. This cleansing effect is suitable also for glass coffee makers and thermos jugs.
– Harris (1968)

Externally, the characteristic 'fizz' of bicarb is what makes it excellent in the bath, for a foot spa or a bath bomb. The abrasion effect can be used as a handy toothpowder that whitens teeth and freshens breath.

Bicarb effectively kills the bacteria that cause body odours, so can offer a ready underarm or foot deodorant. It will also neutralise the venom of bee stings.

The alkalinity of bicarb in a tepid bath helps to soothe sunburn or the irritations of hives, shingles and chickenpox. It has a reputation for easing athlete's foot and acne. Internally, it can be taken safely for bladder infections, and will help clear away crystals of uric acid that can lead to gout.

High protein consumption, typical of western diets, causes the body to produce more acids than bases, which acidifies the blood. Ingesting small amounts of bicarb can help redress this balance, and is beneficial for chronic health problems associated with blood acidity, including arthritis. This is why you will often find it recommended as part of alternative cancer treatments. However, the quickest and most natural way to alkalise the blood is to increase respiration – breathe more deeply or faster. Julie recommends this rather than bicarb to her patients.

The accessible (and cheaply purchased) alkalinity of bicarb has found a more controversial use in supporting athletic performance. As a onetime runner, Matthew read the stories of South African marathon star Arthur Newton who relied on his 'corpse reviver',

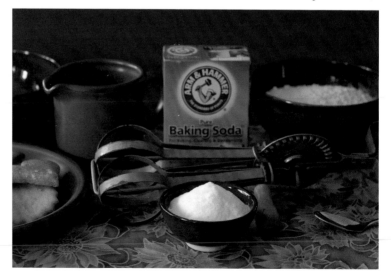

which featured bicarb, in the 1920s. It worked for Newton, who won the gruelling Comrades Marathon five times (see recipe). Bear in mind this was endurance sports in a hot climate, many years before isotonic drinks became available. More recently bicarb has been found beneficial in short, explosive events, like sprinting and swimming, though there are concerns about 'soda doping' or building up excessive sodium levels if taking too much bicarb.

Whether in longer or shorter activity, the bicarb reduces or delays the onset of lactic acid, the body's waste product of tired muscles from physical effort.

Corpse reviver
This mixture is made in a large glass or cup, with 1 tablespoon of **castor sugar** (which dissolves better), ½ teaspoon of **salt** and ¾ teaspoon of **bicarbonate of soda**, to which is added ¼ glass of **water**; mix and top up with **lemonade**. Establish personal preference in dosage by experimentation.

Tooth cleaning powder
Mix equal parts **sea salt** and **bicarbonate of soda**. Store in a jar. To use, tip a small amount into the palm of your hand and dip a damp toothbrush into it. Brush your teeth as normal.

Bicarb bath
Put ½ cupful of **bicarbonate of soda** in the bath.

Bath bombs
Mix in a bowl: 500g (say 1lb) **bicarbonate of soda**, 250g (say ½lb) **citric acid**, ½ teaspoon of **vanilla extract** (or a few drops of essential oil of your choice). Spritz with water from a spray bottle, just enough to make it hold together. Shape into a ball or press into a bath bomb mould. Allow to dry before use.

Deodorant
Place about a teaspoonful of **bicarbonate of soda** in the palm of your hand. Add enough **water** to make a soft paste and rub on your under-arms.

Soda paste
Mix a little **bicarbonate of soda** with enough **water** to make a paste. Apply to chickenpox and shingles, and other blisters and rashes, repeating as needed to relieve pain and itching.

Corpse reviver
- rehydration
- diarrhoea
- endurance sports

Tooth cleaning powder
- routine oral hygiene
- bad breath
- stained teeth

Bicarb bath
- itchy skin
- chickenpox blisters
- shingles
- sunburn
- rashes

Bath bombs
- itchy skin

Deodorant
- body odour

Soda paste
- chickenpox blisters
- shingles
- blisters
- rashes
- insect bites

Cautions for internal use
Do not use bicarb in cases of unknown abdominal pain, or if you have a very full stomach. Avoid if you have high sodium levels. Overuse can result in metabolic imbalances owing to raised sodium levels and increased alkalinity.

Blueberry *Vaccinium corymbosum*

The antioxidants in ripe blueberries are wonderful for the eyes and sight, with a role in delaying the onset of cataract and glaucoma, and macular degeneration. This protective role extends to the bladder and stomach lining, while the dried berries are anti-diarrhoeal. Here is a star attraction in modern supermarkets that also makes a delicious medicine.

**Ericaceae
Heather family**

Description: Both a low, prostrate shrub and a 'high bush' cultivar, which can be 4m (13ft) tall; leaves small and green, some types deciduous and others evergreen; yellow–white flowers followed by berries that turn green, red and finally black as they ripen, with a sweet but tart taste.

Distribution: North American native, also circumpolar and now commercially grown in southern hemisphere.

Related species: *V. corymbosum* is the 'high bush' group and *V. angustifolium* the 'low bush' or wild blueberry group. Other commercially successful *Vacciniums* include cranberry (*V. macrocarpon*) and bilberry (*V. myrtillus*).

Parts used: Fruit and leaves.

When I see, as now, in climbing one of our hills, huckleberry and blueberry bushes bent to the ground with fruit, I think of them as fruits fit to grow on the most Olympian or heaven-pointing hills.
– Thoreau (c. 1850s)

Blueberries are an established fruit favourite in North America and northern Europe, and a relatively new attraction in Britain's supermarkets. Sales of British fresh and frozen blueberries in 2008 were £76 million annually, rising to £300m by 2017.

Hailed in some quarters as a 'superfood', with high antioxidant levels and anthocyanin benefits for the circulation, digestion, urinary system and eye health, these berries have a distinctive sweet–sour taste and rich 'feel-good' texture. Children often love them.

Eaten fresh by themselves, as a flavouring for yogurt, ice cream and fruit smoothies, or cooked in pies and muffins, blueberries are also worth trying as a piquant addition to savoury preparations such as stews and bean dishes. Bred for extra sweetness, as

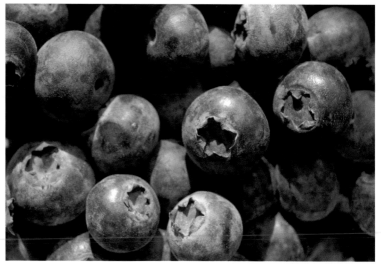

compared with bilberries and cranberries, both members of the same family, cultivated varieties of blueberry, especially market leader Bluecrop, also have larger fruits and heavier yields.

Laborious hand-picking of wild bilberry was always a limitation on its large-scale cultivation in the British Isles. New mechanical harvesting techniques, allied with improvements in taller 'high bush' cultivars, mean that mass supply of blueberries from locally grown fruit is already a reality.

Use blueberries for…

Along with bilberries, cranberries, blackberries and other dark berries, blueberries have a popular reputation for improving night vision and eye health in general.

Scientific research has confirmed and explained this opinion. By their antioxidant action these fruits help prevent 'scavenger' free radicals from breaking down vitamin C and other nutrients in the small blood vessels in the eye. This effectively delays the onset of cataract and glaucoma, and macular degeneration.

Laboratory research also backs up the belief that blueberries are protective in the bladder. The mechanism appears to be that bacteria, including harmful *E. coli*, are prevented from attaching to the bladder walls, thereby cutting chances of infection and cystitis.

In a similar action, bilberries and blueberries work in the stomach lining to produce mucus that is protective against excess digestive acids; this gives the fruits a role in treating gastric ulcers.

Dried blueberries (even more so the leaves) are known to be anti-diarrhoeal, as their astringent tannins and pectin help solidify the stool. Note that the fresh berries help constipation but you need a lot to get a laxative effect.

Broadly, the more bitterness or sourness you allow in your blueberries the better the medicinal result. One hopes the current large-berry cultivars do not lose their astringent edge. And don't swamp your blueberries in sugar and presume your waistline will improve!

Rating your antioxidants

These micro compounds protect the body against oxidation, or cellular damage caused by free radicals. Well-known antioxidants include vitamins C, E and beta-carotene. They have a significant role in maintaining healthy functions in the body, including delaying age degeneration of tissues, as in the retina.

Researchers at the US Department of Agriculture (2007) provided test-tube evidence that wild blueberries had the second highest antioxidant values, after red/blue beans and berries. But a later report by the FDA's Nutrient Data Laboratory (2012) noted mounting evidence that antioxidant capacity of itself had 'no relevance to the effects of specific bioactive compounds including polyphenols on human health'. It is a caution to keep refining our search!

To get the most medicinal benefit from **blueberries**, eat them raw. You can simply munch on a handful a day, put them in fresh fruit salads or fruit smoothies, or preserve them in vinegar.

Blueberry vinegar

Fill a large jar with **fresh blueberries** and pour on **white wine or cider vinegar** to cover them. Leave to macerate for two weeks, then blend or mash. Strain off the liquid and pour into sterile bottles.

Blueberry vinegar
- eye health
- varicose veins
- cystitis
- night vision

Butter & ghee

Butter is a traditional part of the diet in cooler climates. It can be clarified to make ghee, which is almost pure butterfat. Both products can be vehicles for herbs and spices for internal use, and make soothing ointments for the skin.

Butter is produced when cream, the fat from milk, is churned. Most butter is made from cow's milk, but any milk can be used. Goat's butter is now widely available, and is a lighter and more easily digested alternative to cow's butter.

Butter and cream are both an emulsion of fat and water. Cream contains about 40% fat and butter has 80% or more. Once butter has been clarified (as ghee), it is virtually 100% butterfat.

Because many pesticide residues concentrate in commercial fats, we recommend buying organically produced butter if possible.

Butter contains little lactose, so is usually tolerated in moderate amounts by those who are lactose-intolerant. Butter retains very little milk protein, and most people with milk allergies can tolerate some.

Clarified butter or ghee is OK for both groups as it contains neither protein nor lactose.

Butter is more common as a food in cooler climates where it keeps well. In hotter climates it is often clarified by heating it to remove the water and proteins to make ghee, which keeps for long periods without refrigeration.

The ancient Greeks and Romans mainly used olive oil for food, reserving butter for medicinal use as an ointment.

When we were growing up, butter was the first aid remedy for minor burns. Now we know that holding the burn under cold running water for ten minutes is the most effective emergency treatment, but butter may have a secondary role in soothing and protecting the damaged skin afterwards.

Butter versus margarine – which is healthier? Margarine has been sold as a cheaper and healthier alternative, but we vote for butter, in moderation, as it is a more natural product and still tastes better. Margarine is highly processed, contains trans-fatty acids and in many cases has hydrogenated (artificially saturated) fats.

Butter is the only fat that is broken down in the stomach – we needed this as babies when we lived on milk. All other fats wait until they get to the small intestines to be emulsified by bile (stored in the gallbladder) and broken down by pancreatic enzymes. For this reason, people with gallbladder problems may be able to tolerate butterfat better than other fats.

Pastoral peoples use butter as a cosmetic and to protect their skin, often mixing it with powdered resins and other aromatic herbs, and with pigments like red ochre (as do the Himba of Namibia). It is also used as a hair dressing.

Herb butters and honey butter are traditional European combinations, and can be used in cooking and as medicine.

Ghee is very well absorbed by the skin, and makes an excellent base for ointments. It can be used as a massage oil, and makes wonderful face creams as it plumps out the skin, making it look younger. It is the traditional cooking oil in India, though substitutes like mustard oil are cheaper for mass modern use.

A rich pour: home-made ghee

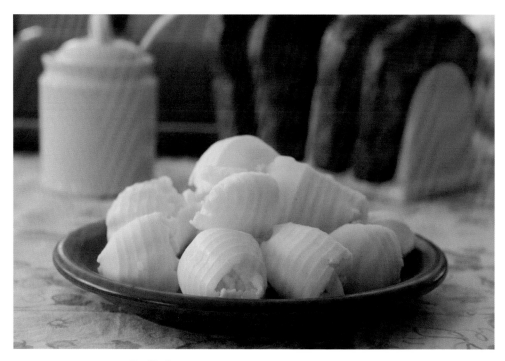

Garlic butter

One of the most delicious ways to take raw garlic for its medicinal properties is in garlic butter.

Squeeze 5 or 6 cloves of **garlic** through a garlic press, or mince finely with a sharp knife and then mash in a mortar and pestle. Mix thoroughly into 250g (8oz) softened **butter**. It keeps well in the refrigerator.

Garlic butter
• infections
• respiratory infections
• fungal infections

Use a dab on hot cooked vegetables or other food. Take more if you are suffering from an infection such as a cold or chest infection. It can also be used externally on the skin as an ointment for fungal infections such as athlete's foot and for bacterial infections such as *Staphylococcus aureus*.

Honey butter
• convalescence
• low energy
• underweight
• dry skin

Alternatives: many other herbs make tasty butters, either singly or in combination. Try thyme, grated lemon peel, lavender, parsley, mint or oregano.

Honey butter

Mix roughly equal amounts of softened **butter** and **honey**, slowly adding the honey to the butter until you have the consistency you want.

Ghee (clarified butter)

To make ghee, melt unsalted **butter** in a saucepan. We usually use four 250g (8oz) packets of butter at a time, but you can make any amount. Recipes for ghee specify unsalted butter, but use ordinary salted butter if that is all you can get. Use organically produced butter if available.

Once the butter has melted, turn up the heat a little and boil the butter on a low to medium heat. Every batch of butter will behave a little differently, so it's difficult to give an exact timing. If the heat is too low, it takes a long time to clarify, if too high the solids on the bottom may burn – so keep an eye on the butter as it boils. Soon the main part of the butter will turn a clear golden colour, with heavy solids settling to the bottom and other impurities forming a foam on the top. Cook it a little longer, until the bottom just starts to caramelise.

Skim off the foam on top of the clarified butter and discard. Pour the clear liquid into jars, leaving any solids behind at the bottom of the pan. We use a fine strainer to catch any solids or bits of foam that we missed.

Ghee remains liquid in a warm climate, but in cooler areas will usually become solid on cooling. It keeps indefinitely without refrigeration.

Clove and black pepper ointment

Crush 2 tablespoons **black peppercorns** and 2 tablespoons **cloves**, and put into a jar with ½ cup of **ghee**. Heat the jar in a pan of hot water for two hours, then strain and pour the ghee into a storage jar or bottle. Once cool it will remain solid in more northerly kitchens.

Ghee lamp

Ghee burns cleanly and brightly, making a lamp that doesn't smoke or smell. Ghee is used in Indian temples instead of oil lamps or candles.

Pour **ghee** into a **small bowl**. If the ghee is solid, you may need to melt it first. Cut a piece of **cotton string** long enough use as a wick – the length needed will depend on the size of your bowl, but it should be long enough to curl a little in the bottom of the bowl. Take a **metal paper clip** and pull the central part upwards to make a stand for one end of the wick. Dip the wick into the ghee to soak it, then place in the bowl with one end supported by the wire near the centre of the bowl. Light with a match. Adjust the wick length as necessary as the lamp burns, and top up with more ghee. Olive oil can be used in the same way.

Ghee
- oleates tissues
- carries herbs deep into the organs
- strengthens brain and nervous system
- supports body heat
- nourishes metabolism
- melts on contact with skin
- readily absorbed

Ghee is a highly effective way of carrying herbs to the deeper tissues of the body.
– Lad (1999)

Clove & black pepper ointment
- muscle aches and pains
- painful joints
- backache
- cold feet
- chilblains

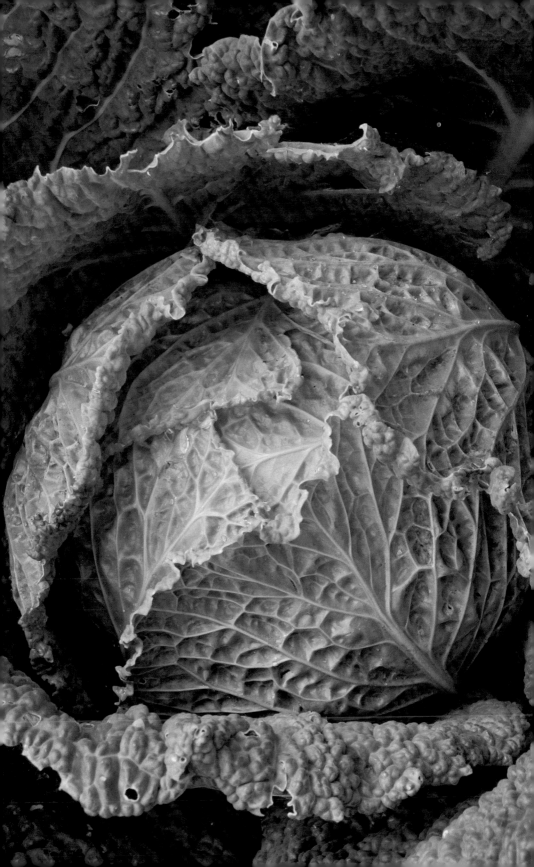

Cabbage *Brassica oleracea*

Cabbage has spent hundreds of years being humble and overlooked, but meanwhile its ready breeding turned the Brassicas into the most successful genus of food plants. Medicinally, it makes an excellent leaf poultice, its juice is cooling and soothing for many conditions, and in fermented form, as sauerkraut, cabbage preserves its vitamins and minerals

Do you have a favourite cabbage moment? Perhaps sadly, we do. It was in the Campo de' Fiori in Rome, one blazing June day. A street trader, a stout middle-aged lady dressed in black, was sporting a hat made of two cabbage leaves, hanging over her ears like a cloche.

It looked amusing – but then we come from a country where men on seaside holidays still tie a knot at each corner of their hanky and put it on their heads as their entire sunscreen programme. How much more eco-friendly and chic to wear a cooling cabbage!

For the Romans of old cabbage was a cure-all. As well as a cooked and pickled vegetable, both wild and domesticated forms were used medicinally. Cabbage juice was taken for headaches, deafness, eye problems, drunkenness, insomnia, colic and stomach ulcers, and cabbage leaf poultices used for aches, swellings and joint pain.

The Romans faded but the cabbage continued to be grown domestically in Europe as a staple food and DIY medicine. Mrs Leyel (1957) relates the story that a young doctor went from his native country to Denmark to start a medical practice but returned on seeing that every garden was well stocked with cabbages. He knew nobody would need his services.

The Dutch were big on cabbage breeding. They also had a secret cabbage remedy. Well, to be fair, it was already known to Pliny, in ancient Rome, but this did not prevent it being called Boerhaave syrup after its Dutch rediscoverer.

This was a powerful domestic treatment for consumption (TB). Red cabbage leaves were pounded by hand, then squeezed through a cloth to collect the juice. Half the weight of the juice was added as honey, and the broth cooked over a gentle heat. The cooking continued until a syrup formed, which was the medicine.

John Parkinson mentioned much the same remedy in 1629, in terms of a 'licking electuary' for 'a Consumption of the lunges'. This

**Brassicaceae
Cabbage family**

The Brassicas have more commercially valued species than any other genus, from roots (such as swedes and turnips), leaves (eg cabbage), flowers (cauliflowers, broccoli) to seeds (mustard, oilseed rape).

Distribution: World-wide in temperate zones.

Related species: Wild or sea cabbage (*Brassica oleracea* subsp. *oleracea*) is the ancestor of cultivated cabbages. Six main groups have emerged in selective breeding: non-heading kales (*acapitata*), heading cabbages (*capitata*), kohlrabi (*gongylodes*), broccoli (*cymosa*), Brussels sprouts (*gemmifera*), and cauliflower (*botyritis*).

Parts used: Leaf.

[cabbage juice is] *a crass and melancholy Juice; yet* Loosening *if but moderately boil'd, if over-much* Astringent *... and therefore seldom eaten raw, excepting by the* Dutch.
– Evelyn (1699)

The fractal world of red cabbage

comprised boiled cabbage stalks with honey and almond milk.

Something similar turned up in twentieth-century North America as 'pectoral syrup' or the 'French formula', a blend of a red cabbage decoction and honey.

In the 1950s, the American doctor Garnet Cheney promoted fresh and unheated cabbage juice as a treatment for duodenal ulcers, naming its special healing quality vitamin U. The name hasn't caught on, but later research has shown that cabbage indeed contains two principles, glutamine and S-methyl methionine, that have known anti-ulcer activity.

In France, the naturopath Dr Valnet (1920–95) called cabbage 'the doctor of the poor', and folk medicine uses repeated the treatments of the Romans of antiquity, with new emphasis on a cabbage decoction for throat infections and whooping-cough.

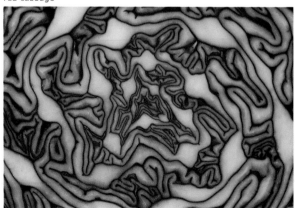

It is to the French that we owe the playful use of cabbage in love-talk: 'mon petit chou' (little cabbage) is sometimes taken to refer to Brussels sprouts. And lest the hanky-wearing British feel neglected in the cabbage love-fest, a Victorian Valentine card offered:

My love is like a cabbage,
Often cut in two.
The leaves I give to others,
The heart I give to you.

Use cabbage for...
If the English swain had kept the leaves for his own use, he would have found a cabbage leaf poultice a good and easy remedy for swellings, aching joints, external ulcers, migraines and bronchitis; or for stings and splinters, swollen eyes, burns and sunburn.

Leaves of any of the cultivated Brassicas will make a good poultice, and equally so the wild members of the wider tribe, like sea kale, rocket or black or white mustard. One caution is that people with sensitive skins may find mustard leaves burning.

Cabbage poultices draw toxins and heat from the affected area, cooling the whole body. Dr Valnet reported cases where this treatment rendered amputation or surgery unnecessary.

Cabbage juice is also effectively cooling, whether made as broth or decoction, and reduces digestive acidity and burning as well as soothes indigestion and constipation. For centuries this remedy has been a specific for stomach and duodenal ulcers.

Cabbage in its fermented form as sauerkraut is a general food remedy for stomach problems of various types. Researchers have shown that the vitamins and minerals in cabbage are preserved most efficiently as sauerkraut.

Additionally, cabbage juice will loosen mucus, allowing expectorants like garlic and ginger to eliminate the mucus more readily. This makes cabbage a good remedy for dry coughs.

James Duke, the American ethnobotanist, rated cabbage his top herb for osteoporosis.

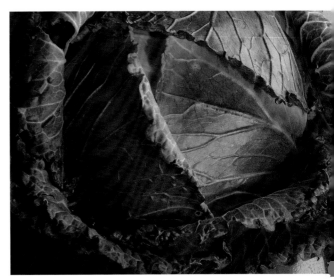

He explained that the boron in cabbage helps raise oestrogen levels in the blood, which is beneficial for bone preservation.

Cabbage poultice

Take some **cabbage** leaves, enough for a double or triple layer. The central stalks can be removed, but it is not vital – in fact, if you are just poulticing something small, like a cut, the stems are the juiciest part.

Pound the cabbage or roll with a rolling pin until the juice begins to emerge. The bruised damp leaves are then applied to the painful place and held in position by a bandage or similar fastening. Keep the poultice on for several hours or overnight and then replace.

Cabbage is particularly good for painful, inflamed scratches and splinters from roses and brambles.

Cabbage juice

Juice a 1 inch (2.5cm) thick slice of a **cabbage**. The juice smells slightly sulphurous but does not taste bad. If you don't have a juicer put the chopped cabbage in a blender with a cup of pure water and blend.

Dose: drink this amount three times daily. The juice can be diluted with water to taste.

Cabbage poultice
- inflammation
- scratches
- splinters
- aching joints
- leg ulcers
- sunburn
- minor burns
- boils
- sore breasts
- lymphoedema

Cabbage juice
- inflammation
- stomach ulcers
- gastric reflux
- aching joints

Cardamom, elachi

Elettaria cardamomum

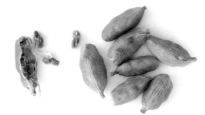

Cardamom is one of the best-known and most expensive Indian spices, with universal appeal as a sweet ingredient in cooking and as a breath-freshener. It is less familiar medicinally, as a digestive stimulant, carminative and respiratory remedy.

**Zingiberaceae
Ginger family**

Description: Tropical evergreen perennial growing to 5m (15ft), with thick rhizomes, long spear-like leaves, white flowers with mauve markings and green three-celled pods, each holding 15–30 black aromatic and pungent seeds, at ground level.

Distribution: Native to S India, now grown in rest of S Asia, China and SE Asia, parts of Africa and Guatemala.

Other cardamoms: There are many related *Amomums* and *Aframomums*, eg Nepalese or greater cardamom (*Amomum subulatum*), Java or round cardamom (*A. compactum*), Chinese cardamom, *sha ren* (*A. villosum* or *A. xanthioides*), and *yi zhi ren* (*Alpinia oxyphylla*), Thai cardamom (*Amomum krarvanh*), Ethiopian or Korarima cardamom, (*Aframomum korarima*), Madagascar cardamom (*Aframomum angustifolium*).

Parts used: Fruit and seeds; essential oil.

Cardamom is a high-price spice, up there on the top table with saffron and vanilla. In India it is called the 'queen of spices' (to pepper's 'king'). Harvesting is time-critical. Cardamom fruits ripen at different times, and the pods are picked green, but have to be just the right green to be dried.

The fruits are usually on low stems at ground level, and each pod yields only 15–30 small seeds. In Guatemala, a leading growing area, producers estimate it takes four pods to fill a quarter of a teaspoon with seeds. Picking is slow and labour-intensive, which is reflected in the market price.

Various cropped plants claim cardamom in their name, but the highest market status is given to *Elettaria cardamomum*, which yields the elliptical lime-green pods many of us are familiar with. This is native to south India, on both the Mysore and Malabar sides, and more recently has found excellent growing conditions in Guatemala and East Africa. The Latin *Elettaria* was taken from the local Malabar name.

Other cardamoms, sometimes collectively called and dismissed as 'false cardamom', are occasionally used to adulterate the valuable south Indian crop, though they do differ visually and have their own limited provenance in trade. They tend to be browner or even black, and can be larger and rounder in appearance.

The trade in cardamom is ancient: the pharaonic Egyptians valued Indian cardamom as a breath cleanser, and the Greeks knew and had named both the *cardamomum* and inferior *amomum* types by the 4th century BC.

The Romans kept up the trade, using cardamom in sweet/sour sauces to aid digestion, while in the Middle Ages cardamom was an important ingredient in hippocras (mulled sweetened wine) and was already used as an aphrodisiac in Islamic cultures.

People have always appreciated the sweet and evocative aroma of cardamom. This arises from the volatile oils of the fruits, which combine eucalyptus, camphor and lemon notes in a unique blend that is uplifting and generous to the nose, the breath and digestion. The Indian cardamom often has a high eucalyptus level, while Nepalese and Chinese varieties tend to contain more camphor.

Cardamom is a good mixer: it is superb in coffee, as a tea or chai; it is used both in curries and cakes, not to mention ice cream. The powder is known as *elachi* in India, which goes into popular milk shakes and sweets.

Cardamom combines well with other spices and herbs, and can mask unpleasant tastes in digestive remedies; it has a long use in perfumery and cosmetics, often in essential oil form.

A word on storage: you really can't improve on Nature, as the pods effectively seal in the aroma, which the powdered form loses in a few days. Keep your pods in a dry bottle in the dark until needed, then grind electrically or in a pestle and mortar. It is fiddly but easy enough to pick out the seed cases from your hand-ground mixture, and if you are grinding for filter coffee, use the cases too.

Cardamom has no marked drug interactions, and is safe for babies as well as the very sick. The only downside is for people with photosensitive skin who may find that handling cardamom with bare hands in any quantity can lead to contact dermatitis.

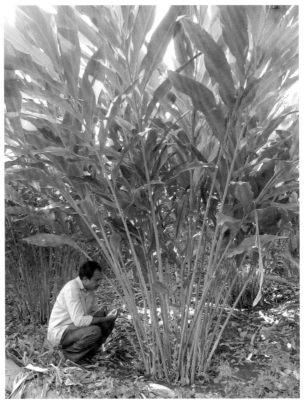

A cardamom farmer in Kerala checks the ripening pods

Cardamom pods are like Christmas trees. The greener and bigger they are, the more they're worth.
–Dr Luis Pedro Torrebiarte, president of the Cardamom Exporters' Association of Guatemala (1997)

[cardamoms] *form part of the furniture of the sireh* [silver spice box] *of a person of distinction.*
– Stamford Raffles (1817)

Use cardamom for...

As a member of the ginger family – and even though it is the fruit that is used rather than the rhizomes, as in ginger and turmeric, say – cardamom is an excellent digestive stimulant. In Ayurveda and Chinese medicine it has long been a specific for weak and cold digestion, which 'kindles the digestive fire', including increasing the appetite.

Continuing the theme of stimulation, cardamom boiled in

milk and honey is an Ayurvedic treatment for male impotence or premature ejaculation.

Cardamom is a carminative, ie helps settle bloating and intestinal gas in the form of flatulence, indigestion and hiccups. It is palatable to children suffering from vomiting, and it particularly settles milk reflux.

Cardamom is also useful in respiratory issues, as you might expect from a spice that contains both eucalyptus and camphor. A cardamom tea mix with cinnamon, clove and pepper is useful for lung problems. Cardamom can also soothe a sore throat, help cut mucus, and as an antispasmodic will ease coughing fits or asthma attacks, and reduce hoarseness. A daily cardamom gargle is an

Indian kitchen remedy to prevent or minimise the onset of influenza.

Cardamom is uplifting, and helps clear the head in cases of stress headaches, and those caused by indigestion. It makes the mouth feel sweeter and restores the taste. Chew a pod of cardamom for fresh breath, and you have one of the oldest and simplest herbal recipes in the world. It was known to Egyptians, Indians and Chinese of three thousand years ago, as their written records show.

For ethnobotanist James Duke cardamom was a top remedy for stale breath, the essential oils destroying the mouth bacteria that cause the problem. It will also reduce the haze of alcohol or garlic on the breath. The Romans of old knew this, and it still works.

... one of the best and safest digestive stimulants.
– Frawley & Lad (2001)

These aromatic seed pods are filled with soothing, relaxing and antispasmodic essential oils. A premium digestive aid and mucus reducer.
– Pole (2008)

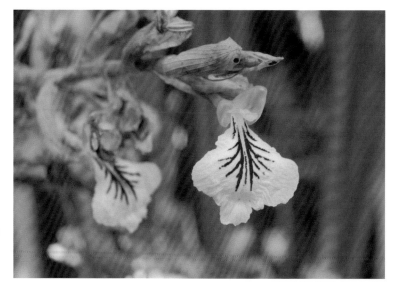

Cardamom flowers

Cardamom milk

Mix 1 teaspoon **cardamom powder** and 250ml (about ½ pt) fresh **milk** in your blender. The cardamom neutralises the mucus-forming property of the milk, giving a 'clean' taste that children love.

Fresh cardamom pods

Elachi energiser

Blend ½ cup each of **pine nuts** and **almonds**, a small **banana** and 1½ cups **oat milk** with 1 tablespoon **cardamom powder**. Add honey, salt and vanilla to taste. Makes enough for two or three drinks, and will keep in fridge for up to three days.

Cardamom pudding

Measure 2 tablespoons **arrowroot** into a bowl and mix with a little cold milk to form a thin paste. Heat in a saucepan 2 cups **milk**, 1 teaspoon **cardamom powder** and 2 tablespoons **sugar**. Stir into the arrowroot paste until thick and add 1 teaspoon **vanilla extract**. It is ready to serve almost at once, or you can allow to cool if you prefer.

Cardamom electuary

Grind in an electric grinder until smooth: 3 tablespoons **pine nuts**, 3 tablespoons **raisins**, 3 tablespoons runny **honey**, 1 tablespoon **whisky**, ½ teaspoon **cardamom powder** and ¼ teaspoon **cinnamon powder**.

Cardamom syrup

Crush 2 tablespoons of **cardamom pods**. Put in a saucepan with 2 cups **water** and simmer gently with the lid on for about half an hour.

Strain out the cardamom and return the liquid to the pan. Add 1 cup **sugar** and bring to the boil, boiling until reduced by about half and the syrup is beginning to thicken. Add the juice of half a **lemon**, bring to the boil again, then remove from the heat and bottle.

Dose: 1 teaspoonful as needed for sore throats, dry tickly coughs and laryngitis.

Cardamom coffee

Add a few pods of **cardamom** to your **coffee beans** when you grind them, or if you don't have a grinder add ¼ teaspoon cardamom powder to your pre-ground coffee. Cardamom not only tastes great with coffee, but it reduces the negative effects of coffee, such as the jitteriness it sometimes causes, without affecting the general stimulatory effect.

Cardamom milk
- convalescence
- digestion
- minimises mucus

Elachi energiser
- convalescence
- weakness
- exercise

Cardamom pudding
- convalescence
- weak digestion

Cardamom electuary
- coughs
- sore throats
- laryngitis

Cardamom syrup
- coughs
- sore throats
- hoarseness
- weak digestion
- colds

Cardamom coffee
- stimulating without making you feel scattered and jittery

Carrot *Daucus carota*, subsp. *sativus*

Apiaceae (Umbelliferae) Carrot family

Description: Biennial, erect and wiry, to 1m (3ft), tall; white flowers in flat umbels that curve inwards when ripe, like a bird's nest (an old name for the plant).

Distribution: Temperate zones of Europe, Asia, Africa; naturalised in North America and most parts of the world.

Wild carrot: Wild carrot or Queen Anne's lace (*D. carota*, var. *carota*) has white flowers with a purplish-red centre. The name comes from a story that Queen Anne once cut her finger when making lace.

Parts used: Root, leaves, seeds.

Sowe Carrets in your Gardens, and humbly praise God for them, as for a singular and great blessing.
– Gardiner (c. 1599)

If cigarettes are cancer sticks, carrots are anti-cancer sticks. ... Even if you don't quit smoking, you should still be munching on carrots.
– Duke (1997)

Carrot is a familiar vegetable with a folk medicine reputation for improving night vision and smoothing wrinkles; it is a mild, nourishing food for infants with diarrhoea and soothes the digestive tract. Claims studied in clinical trials include reducing lung cancer risk and assistance in asthmatic conditions.

The carrot is a triumph of cultivation. Beginning with a small, bitter, wild, annual plant, breeders over centuries have created a sturdy, fleshy and sweet biennial that is one of the best-selling vegetables in the world.

The modern carrot is packed with sugars and starches, vitamins A and C, and many minerals. It is a well-bred distance from its wiry, bitter-tasting progenitor, yet can still revert to the genetic predecessor if left untended.

The original growing region is thought to be the Hindu Kush area of central Asia, where carrots have forked roots and tend to be blue or red, from the anthocyanins they contain. Modern orange-hued carrots derive from European, particularly Dutch, breeding efforts in the sixteenth and later centuries. These plants are typified by undivided orange or yellow taproots rich in beta-carotene.

Carrots are versatile, being tasty raw or cooked. Naturally sweet, they are used in cakes and desserts as well as savoury dishes.

Use carrots for...

Past herbalists often used wild carrot seed as a diuretic and as a specific for urinary stones. The seed also has an old reputation as a 'morning-after' contraceptive. These properties are less evident in the cultivated form, which however has other benefits.

Beta-carotene is a naturally occurring precursor for carotene, or vitamin A. Modern, and particularly organic, carrots thus work on bodily functions influenced by carotene, including the kidneys, lungs, eyes and skin.

Beta-carotene is an antioxidant that appears to locate and destroy carcinogens in the lungs and pancreas. This includes tobacco residues, so linking carrots to lung cancer treatments. The ancient Greeks knew that carrots supported the respiratory system, giving wild carrots to wheezy horses. We'd now add that asthmatic humans benefit from regular carrot intake.

And yes, research does support folk wisdom that carrots improve

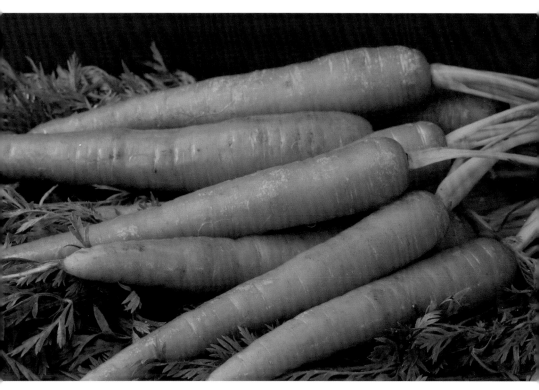

the eyes, including night vision and prevention of cataracts, from the vitamin A link. Keeping vitamin A levels high maintains skin elasticity, meaning that eating carrots might delay wrinkles.

Two kinds of carrot oil are produced commercially. Carrot seed oil is an essential oil distilled from wild carrot seed, while the oil from the root is a macerated oil used in skincare products and suntan lotions. Don't just discard your carrot tops either – they are high in potassium, and can be added to broths, or small amounts minced and added to salads. Julie's father remembered his mother using a traditional childhood pinworm treatment, grated carrot as a one-day mono-diet. Finally, a baby or infant suffering with diarrhoea can often stomach a soothing purée of carrots to replace lost nutrients.

... the elusive 'Carrot factor', despite current infatuation with one carrot essence – betacarotene – is quite likely the whole carrot itself.
– Carper (1988)

Carrot oil
Grate two **carrots** and measure the grated amount. Add an equal volume of **olive oil** (or coconut oil) and fry gently until the carrots are soft and the oil has turned orange. Strain and bottle the oil.

Carrot lassi
Blend equal parts of **fresh carrot juice** and **natural live yogurt**, and season to taste with **sea salt** and **cumin** or **coriander** powder.

Carrot oil
- chapped skin
- dry skin
- sunburn
- sun damage
- eczema
- itchy skin

Carrot lassi
- heat
- weak digestion
- after antibiotics

Celery

Apium graveolens var. *dulce*

Apiaceae (Umbelliferae) Carrot family

Description: Biennial, up to 1m (40in) high, with upright, slender multiple stems, white umbels and brown seeds (fruits).

Distribution: Wild celery is found on marshland (celery is actually a marshwort) and near sea coasts, in Europe and temperate Asia; introduced to North America.

Related plants: Celeriac is a variety of celery (*A. graveolens* var. *rapaceum)* bred for its bulbous root. Alexanders (*Smyrnium olusatrum*) is a wild hedgerow plant with a celery taste, flowering in early spring.

Parts used: Seeds, stems, leaves, roots.

The roots operate by urine, and are very good in fits of the stone or gravel, … A strong decoction made of them is the most effectual preparation. The seeds are of a warm carminative nature; they disperse wind in the stomach and bowels, and operate more powerfully by urine than any other part of the plant.
– Meyrick (1789)

The whitish celery we use in our salads, stews and soups is literally a pale shadow of its dark green and bitter wild ancestor, but it retains medicinal benefits. Celery and its seed is an important remedy in treating sore, swollen and stiff joints and muscles – for arthritis, rheumatism and gout. Its diuretic action also helps with high blood pressure and water retention.

Like many other umbellifers, wild celery has an ancient history of use. Its leaves were woven into funerary garlands in ancient Egypt, and celery oil was used to massage swollen, arthritic limbs.

Celery is mentioned in Homer's *Odyssey*, his '*selinon'* giving the English common name. Greeks and Romans of classical times used it as a bitter flavour in cooking and the seeds as a condiment. Wild celery, *ache des marais* or *fruit de céleri*, is still favoured in France. The first name comes into English as 'smallage', the old name for celery.

Given the antiquity of its wild use, only relatively recently did celery take on its modern cultivated form. From the sixteenth century Italian farmers experimented successfully with earthing up celery stems to deprive them of light and blanch them. This would yield both table celery, with less bitter white stems (hence the variety name, *dulce*), and a swollen-root mild form, celeriac (var. *rapaceum*). Some modern varieties are self-blanching.

Celery has long been used as an aphrodisiac. In eighteenth-century France Madame de Pompadour, mistress of Louis XV, popularised a celery soup, adorned with truffles, that she called 'un régime un peu échauffant' (somewhat stimulating).

Use celery for…

All parts of celery are medicinal, notably the seeds. It is rich in mineral salts, which have an alkalising effect in the body, and essential oils (eg apiol, which gives the celery smell). These combine to break up solidified deposits of uric acid in the joints and help eliminate the waste via the bloodstream and kidneys, also increasing the flow of urine.

The old herbals recommended celery decoctions for kidney stones and 'obstructions of the viscera'. Wild celery is powerful enough to do this, though modern celery stalks are more modest diuretics.

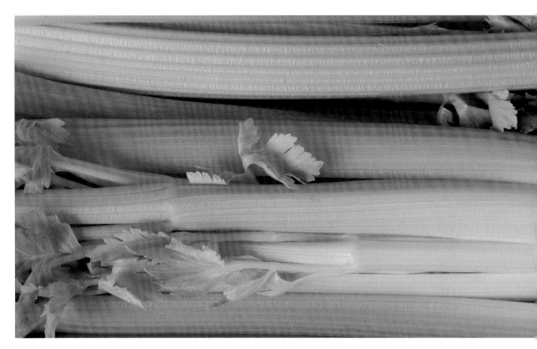

Celery seed remains 'official' as a diuretic in the most recent *British Herbal Pharmacopoeia* (1996). Its effect contributes to reducing high blood pressure (hypertension) and water retention (oedema).

Celery seed is more warming and aromatic than the vegetable, which is cooling and cleansing. Both are effective in treating arthritis, rheumatism and gout. Herbalists also use celery as a nervine for depression, when accompanied by 'nervous restlessness' or 'fidgets'.

Eating celery regularly can also help prevent cramp, and relieves fibromyalgia. Julie's grandmother ate celery every day, and gave it credit for the fact that she had no arthritis though she lived into her nineties – she may well have been right. Dieters will know already that celery is a good filler snack and refreshes the breath.

... a key remedy in European herbal medicine in the treatment of arthritic and rheumatic problems. – Chevallier (2007)

Celery seed
• arthritis
• gout
• rheumatism
• high blood pressure
• oedema

Celery seed decoction
• arthritis
• gout
• rheumatism

Caution: The seeds (being much stronger than the vegetable) should not be used in pregnancy as they can stimulate the uterus.

Celery seed
Simply chew ½ teaspoonful of **celery seed** daily.

Celery seed decoction
Simmer two tablespoons of **celery seed** in a cup of **water**, until reduced to half a cup. Cool and take a teaspoonful twice a day.

Chilli/cayenne pepper

Capsicum annuum, var. *annuum; C. frutescens*

**Solanaceae
Nightshade family**

Description:
Annuals or short-lived
perennials, to 1.5m
(5ft) tall, with oval
leaves, small, bell-like
white flowers followed
by pendant or upright,
conical or spherical red,
yellow or green fruits.

Distribution:
Indigenous to Mexico
and northern South
America, now grown
in many tropical and
subtropical areas,
especially Africa and
South Asia.

Similar species:
Capsicums have five
main cultivar groups
(see box, p52), the
largest being *C.
annuum,* var. *annuum.*
Over 1700 capsicum
varieties are grown.

Parts used: Ripe fruit
is eaten or ground
into chilli and cayenne
pepper powder.

*... there is also plenty
of aji [chilli], which is
their pepper, which is
more valuable than
[black] pepper, and
all the people eat
nothing else, it being
very wholesome. Fifty
caravels might be
annually loaded with it
[to take to Spain].
– Christopher
Columbus, from ship's
log, 14 January 1492,
off Hispaniola*

**Chilli powder and cayenne are ground
from ripe, dried fruits of capsicums, whose heat depends on the
amount of capsaicin they contain – none in bell peppers and a
lot in habañeros. A food preservative in the tropics, chillis have
plentiful vitamin C and are an unparalleled heating stimulant
for colds and 'flu, and circulatory and digestive problems.**

It is well known that Christopher Columbus failed to find the New World spices he so desired, such as a source of black pepper. But he stumbled upon something that would prove even more valuable in the long run – chillies.

These were a mainstay of the New World diet, a medicinal remedy, and central to ritual and sacred tradition. Columbus saw none of that and also managed to misname the plants, beginning a confusion that still persists. Still he discovered that the amazing heat of his 'pimiento' transferred to cultivars that would produce fruit in areas with hot summers.

Chillies spread rapidly in Spanish and Portuguese lands and trading areas, reaching Italy in 1526 and Hungary, then part of Turkey, by 1569, as paprika. Unfortunately for Columbus and others (who stood to gain one-tenth of the proceeds), because the new spice adapted to European and Asian conditions it removed the prospect of a trade monopoly, as there had been for spices with limited growing areas such as cloves and black pepper.

But there was to be ultimate justification for Columbus, and in time to celebrate the 500th year of his first voyage. The writer and 'medicine hunter' Chris Kilham notes that in 1992, for the first time, sales of chilli (in salsa) in the USA exceeded those of tomatoes (in ketchup). As Kilham put it, 'America has traded her favor of sweet and tangy table sauce for the licking flames of chile fever'.

Over thirty capsicums have been identified, with five leading cultivar groups. The main group, *Capsicum annuum,* var. *annuum,* includes bell or 'red' peppers with very little heat, but plentiful nutrients and carotenoids, and also hotter types, like chilli. The longer they are left to ripen and the greater the intensity of the sun the more capsaicin is formed and the hotter they get.

The heat – or, to be precise, the number of times chilli needs to

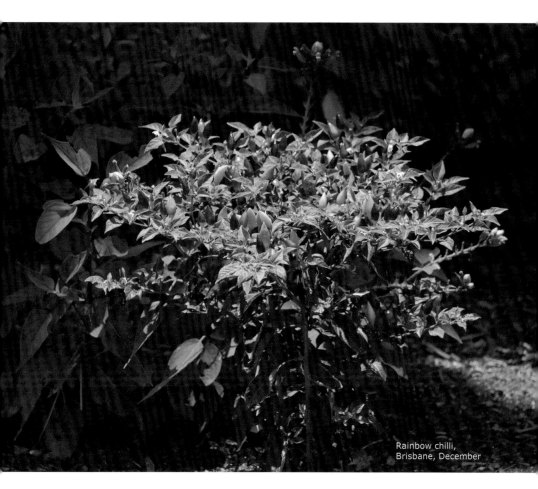
Rainbow chilli,
Brisbane, December

be diluted in water to remove its heat – is calculated in Scoville Heat Units (SHU). This scale also recently celebrated a centenary, being first formulated in 1912.

To give a few examples, bell or sweet peppers rate 0–100 SHU; jalapeño and cayenne are 2500–4000 SHU; tabasco is 60,000–80,000; and habañero is 100,000–300,000. These are seriously hot, for 'mouth surfers' only, so let's cool off a moment and look at the benefits of the chilli, cayenne or tabasco on our kitchen shelves.

Use chilli/cayenne pepper for…

When Matthew was living in South Africa, before he met Julie, he intuitively discovered one of the therapeutic effects of chilli. He was doing a lot of distance running at the time, and found that when you are endurance fit you are prone to colds, blocked sinuses and respiratory problems.

He wanted the clearing heat of chilli but could not take enough of it in food. Tomato juice was the carrier he needed, with two teaspoons of powder to a cup of

People talk of the 'spice of life'. What spice do they mean? … The best candidate is cayenne, as one tiny pinch spices up the whole system.
– Hedley & Shaw (1996)

As a general stimulant and corrector of circulatory problems it has no equal. I find it to be the single most useful cardiovascular remedy in my practice.
– Wood (1997)

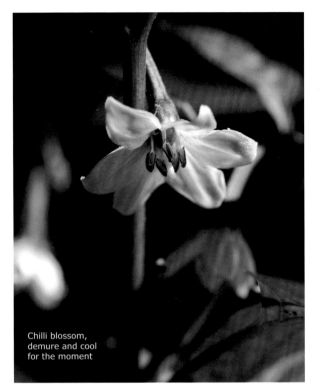

Chilli blossom,
demure and cool
for the moment

juice making a palatable mixture. As a winter warmer that supports the immune system and lifts the spirits, thus lightening depressive moods, this is a simple recipe that we can still recommend.

Chilli has well-established cardiovascular benefits in getting the blood to the extremities (we all know how soon our face goes red when we eat a hot pepper), which is good news for sufferers of Raynaud's and atherosclerosis.

Chilli clears the head and lungs and, not surprisingly, works on the digestion as such, being remedial in cases of indigestion, nausea and loss of appetite. It has plentiful vitamin C and is also known to kill certain stomach nematodes.

In older herbals, such as *King's Dispensatory* of 1898, cayenne tincture with orange peel tincture is extolled for tackling alcoholism and delirium tremens. Present-day herbalists no longer prescribe this, but chilli retains a value at the extreme end of the healing spectrum. One advocate was herbalist and naturopath Dr Christopher (1909–83): 'Cayenne is the purest and most certain stimulant, used medicinally and also as a condiment.'

Dr Christopher recommended ½ teaspoonful in a little warm water as an emergency hot infusion after heart attack, and chilli powder to pack open wounds, even when these were down to the bone.

Chilli con-fusion

Columbus began the confusion by naming the plants he found in 1492 '(red) pepper' (*pimiento*), for there is no botanical connection between the capsicum genus and black pepper, *Piper nigrum*.

Pimiento is now used mainly to describe the sweet or bell peppers, which are vegetables rather than spices, used in salads or cooked. *Pimento* is another name for allspice (a myrtle).

The capsicums are part of the Solanaceae (nightshade family), so are related to tomatoes and potatoes. All capsicums are chillies, with 'pepper' an optional add-on term. Alternative spellings, insisted on in some regions (especially the US), are chili and chile.

There are five main capsicum cultivars:
• *Capsicum annuum*, the largest group, includes paprika, bell peppers, cayenne, jalapeños and chiltepin
• *Capsicum frutescens*: tabasco, Thai and bird peppers
• *Capsicum chinense*, the hottest peppers: naga, habañero and Scotch bonnet
• *Capsicum pubescens*: rocoto peppers
• *Capsicum baccatum*: aji peppers.

'Chili powder' can be the ground-up powder of any type of chilli or a mixture of several. In parts of the US, 'chile powder' is the spice blend that goes into chilli con carne, and also contains cumin, clove and garlic.

Hot pain-relieving oil

Put ½ cup of extra virgin **olive oil** in a small jam jar. Add 3 tablespoons of whatever hot spices you have to hand, eg **chopped chillies**, crushed **mustard seed**, grated fresh **ginger** and crushed **garlic**. If you only have dried powdered spices use 5 teaspoons: chilli powder, mustard powder, ginger powder and black pepper. Put the lid on the jar and shake well. Put it in a warm place to infuse – a sunny windowsill works well. If you need to use the oil straightaway, heat the jar in a pan of hot water.

Cold-banishing soup

For each person, heat 2 cups of **water or vegetable stock** in a saucepan. Add 1 **onion**, finely diced, 1 or 2 teaspoons of chopped **chillies** and 1 or 2 tablespoons of grated fresh **ginger**. Add 2 cloves crushed **garlic**. If you have **chives or spring onions**, chop and add. Halve and slice a couple of **shiitake** or other **mushrooms**. Add any other vegetables you like, eg chopped red or green pepper, some peas, watercress or cabbage. Simmer gently for 15 minutes. Season to taste with sea salt, soy sauce or miso.

Hot pain-relieving oil
- muscle aches & pains
- sore joints
- arthritis
- backache
- sprains and strains
- chilblains
- cold feet
- ganglions

Cold-banishing soup
- chills
- colds
- 'flu
- coughs
- poor circulation

Caution: constitutionally 'hot' people may find chilli too heating.

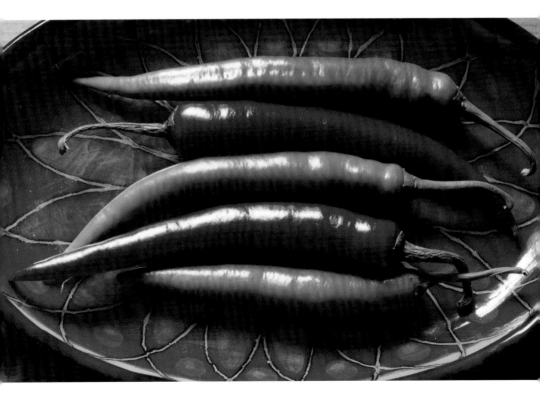

Chilli/cayenne pepper

Chocolate whisk, vanilla pods, cocoa nibs and cocoa powder with a Mexican Garden of Eden candelabrum

Chocolate *Theobroma cacao*

Chocolate, as any chocoholic knows, is a mood enhancer. It is perhaps the food that people who love it get most passionate about. Its Latin name even means 'food of the gods'.

There are good reasons why chocolate has this effect on people – it contains feel-good chemicals and enhances brain activity, and it makes us feel like we're in love. What could be better?

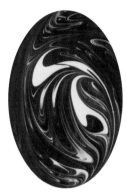

Chocolate was fundamental to the pre-Colomban civilisations of South and Central America where the beans were so valuable they were used as currency. This was literally money growing on trees.

Columbus encountered cocoa in 1502 when he captured a canoe containing a cargo of cacao beans, but it was not until the Spanish met Moctezuma in the Aztec capital of Tenochtitlan in 1519 that reports of chocolate use began to sift back to Europe. Moctezuma was reported to drink 50 cups (from a golden goblet) a day of a specially prepared foamy drink called Xocolatl. Mayan nobles visiting Spain in 1544 introduced the court to drinking chocolate.

The Spanish guarded their secret, closely – when English pirates captured a Spanish treasure galleon, and found bags of what looked like sheep dung on board, which they threw overboard in digust, they had no idea that cocoa beans were worth more than gold.

London's first chocolate house opened in 1657. Chocolate houses rapidly became the fashionable place for wealthy gentlemen to meet. White's, the oldest London club still extant, began in 1693 as a chocolate house.

Chocolate was mainly served as a drink, though it was incorporated into cakes in England. The first chocolate bar was commercially produced by Frys in England in 1847. Milk chocolate was invented by a Swiss chocolatier and first marketed in 1875.

To make chocolate, the beans are usually roasted – although raw cocoa is readily available now for making your own artisan version. The beans are finely ground to produce cocoa mass, which is split under high pressure into cocoa butter and cocoa powder. Making commercial chocolate is a complex art, involving processes of fine grinding, conching and tempering. Sugar, lecithin and often milk solids are added.

The divine drink, which builds up resistance and fights fatigue. A cup of this precious drink permits a man to walk for a whole day without food.
– attributed to Moctezuma (1519)

Chocolate contains small amounts of the chemical **phenylethylamine** (PEA), which is a mild mood elevator. This is the chemical our brain produces in response to feelings of joy and love.

Chocolate has also been shown to boost **serotonin** levels. Serotonin is a neurotransmitter produced by the body, which acts, among other functions, as our brain's own antidepressant.

Chocolate lifts **endorphin** levels in the brain. Endorphins are what flood the brain during times of peak physical exertion, creating a sensation of permeating bliss, such as the fabled 'runner's high'.

Dark chocolate and cocoa contain high levels of **flavonoids**, which are powerful antioxidants in the body, mopping up many free radicals and slowing age-ing. Research has shown that the flavonoids in chocolate and cocoa encourage the improvement of vascular wall health and better functioning of blood vessels.

Milk binds to antioxidants, inhibiting their absorption, so dark chocolate and Aztec-style cocoa without milk have most benefit.

A Mayo Clinic report suggests that moderate amounts of dark chocolate may be used to reduce the risk of blood clots and platelet formation in the arteries that can lead to stroke and heart attacks. Another reason to eat chocolate!

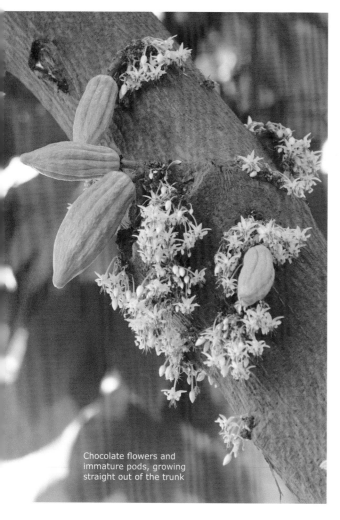

Chocolate flowers and immature pods, growing straight out of the trunk

Use chocolate for...

Chocolate makes you feel happier, and not just because it tastes so good. One reason is that it melts at almost the same temperature as human body heat (34–38°C), giving it the special quality chocolatiers call 'mouthfeel'.

Cocoa is a naturally high source of magnesium, which partly explains why it has been shown to benefit people with chronic fatigue syndrome. Blood flow to the brain increases when chocolate is eaten.

Cocoa and dark chocolate are mildly stimulating, from the alkaloids caffeine and theobromine, but the energy boost from milk chocolate probably owes more to its sugar content.

Cough research has shown theobromine to be more effective than codeine, currently considered the best cough medicine, in suppressing persistent coughs. It works by reducing vagus nerve activity in the upper respiratory tract, but does not cause drowsiness, as codeine does.

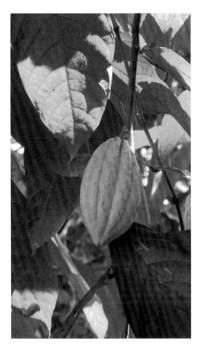

Mature pod, turning from green to yellow

The Maya have given us maize, amaranth, pumpkins, kidney beans, avocadoes, papaya, guava, chilli peppers, chicle, vanilla, tobacco and dahlias as well as chocolate.
– Sams & Fairley (2008)

People no longer remember that Cocoa is a powerful, sacred, medicinal and darned tasty plant. The chocolate of mass appeal in our country [USA] is but a shadow of true Cocoa, being mostly refined sugar, and even the gourmet hot cocoas sold at exorbitant prices abound in artificial flavors and ingredients.
– McDonald (2009)

Theobroma tincture
Put **cocoa nibs** (small chunks of cocoa bean) or **cocoa powder** in a jar and pour in enough **vodka** to cover. The nibs are better than the powder as it is easier to strain, but powder is more readily available. Leave for about 2 weeks, then strain through a jelly bag or fine strainer, and bottle. The medicinal dose is 1 teaspoon 3 times a day, but you can also sweeten to taste and use as a liqueur simply because it tastes good.

Options: add **rosewater** or **rose glycerite** for hormone balance or **cola nut tincture** to make it more grounding, tonic and strengthening.

Aztec cocoa
This is our own modern approximation of the original drinking chocolate enjoyed by the Aztecs.

Using a heaped teaspoon of **cocoa powder** per cup of water in a saucepan, bring it to the boil and whisk until the cocoa has mixed well. Remove from heat, add a pinch of **cayenne powder** (chilli powder) and ½ teaspoon of **vanilla extract**. Add honey to taste.

Theobroma tincture
• nerve tonic
• depression
• depletion

Aztec cocoa
• nerve tonic
• depression
• depletion
• circulation to brain

Cinnamon sticks in close-up look like pillars of an ancient temple

Cinnamon *Cinnamonum zeylanicum, C. verum*

Cinnamon has been a valued spice of trade for several millennia, often confused with and adulterated by its cousin cassia. Known more as a cooking spice these days, cinnamon's medicinal benefits are both traditional (for digestive and respiratory problems, viral infections and stopping bleeding) and more cutting-edge (for treating type-2 diabetes, candida and reducing cholesterol).

Cinnamon is one of the ancient spices, being traded and used in all the historic civilisations of the Middle East, India and China. Its source in Sri Lanka (recalled in the species name *zeylanicum*) was a secret well kept by Arab and Phoenician merchants who controlled the trade until the western European nations began expanding their maritime empires and sought out the places where exotic valuable spices originated.

The 'true' cinnamon, *Cinnamonum verum*, of Sri Lanka has a shadow, the 'bastard' or Chinese cinnamon, *C. cassia*, the cassia plant, from China and Burma. The spice in both cases is the scraped inner bark and the essential oil distilled from the bark, leaf and root. Cassia is rougher, hotter and heavier in taste and aroma, although its pharmacological range is similar to true cinnamon's.

The two types resemble each other enough to be confusing, particularly in powder form, and charges of adulteration have probably accompanied the trade for at least five thousand years.

Perhaps it's simply best to enjoy the true or less true forms as beautiful and uplifting spices, redolent of the Orient and good on toast and cooked apples, and spiced winter drinks! Cinnamon can be used in sweet or in savoury dishes, making it a very versatile cooking ingredient.

In each case the powder loses its savour in storage, though it remains potent if kept in glass and preferably in the dark, for up to a year.

Cinnamon has 'secularised' and lost its 'magic' status over its long history. It was an anointing oil in the Old Testament and for Holy Roman Emperors. It was so precious in ancient Rome that the emperor Nero burnt a year's supply on his wife's funeral pyre, an extravagance to signify the depth of his loss.

Its drying qualities meant that cinnamon was the only spice used in mummifications in pharaonic Egypt; even here cassia might be used as a substitute. It was burned then for incense, and still is.

**Lauraceae
Laurel family**

Description: Attractive evergreen tree, around 10m (30–35ft) tall, with pale thick bark, shiny and leathery green leaves, small whitish flowers and black fruit.

Distribution: Native of Sri Lanka, grown commercially there on hillsides and around the Indian Ocean, in China and Indonesia.

Related species: Up to 100 related species give tree bark that is used in cooking and medicinally; the main commercial species are *Cinnamonum cassia, C. aromaticum* or *C. iners* (cassia), *C. camphora* (camphor tree).

Parts used: Inner bark, dried as quills and powder; bark, leaf and root distilled for an essential oil.

Cinnamon rolls, known as 'cinnamon snails' in Denmark

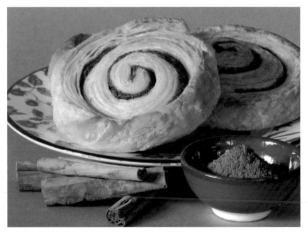

Use cinnamon for...

Cinnamon is a warm and drying spice, which works on the lungs, digestion, circulation and the reproductive system. It is pleasant and mildly stimulating, like cardamom, but less fiery than ginger. It combines well with both, and with other spices, making bitterness easier to swallow.

Cinnamon is good for clearing mucus from the lungs and sinuses, hence is effective for coughs and colds. A head cold can be improved by simply chewing on a cinnamon stick. Think cinnamon for staph infections. It is an excellent spice to give to older people in winter to help them fight off seasonal infections.

Boil up some sticks in water to make a tasty decoction that promotes sweating and will contribute to breaking a fever by eliminating toxins through the skin. Diluted wine or a fruit cordial also make good carriers. As cinnamon powder becomes mucilaginous and gloopy when heated with liquids, we don't find this as inviting as using the whole or crumbled-up quills.

Cinnamon is equally good for improving digestive problems, warming you gently when you are cold and chilled, over-tired and low in resistance or have shivers. The ecclesiastical writer Venerable Bede (AD 673–735) took the trouble to record that cinnamon and cassia were 'very effective in curing disorders of the guts'.

Its tannins making it somewhat astringent, cinnamon is a good treatment for nausea, and will soothe diarrhoea by reducing fluid loss while also helping calm the eruptions of flatulence and colic.

Children will usually tolerate up to a teaspoon of cinnamon powder in hot, sweetened milk as a remedy for diarrhoea and tummy upsets. For adults with the same conditions, use more cinnamon in the formula, according to taste.

Another action of cinnamon is to warm up the extremities by helping the blood circulation move more freely. This relieves pain in arthritic joints and the lower back. Night urination (nocturia) is moderated in a similar manner.

Cinnamon also nourishes the reproductive system in both sexes. In women it can be used for disturbed periods or cramps and cysts. The mucilage helps dry up excessive uterine bleeding after childbirth (a so-called haemostyptic). For men in India it is used for treating impotence. As late as the eighteenth century in England newly weds were given a 'posset' for the marriage bed. The posset mixed wine, milk, egg yolk, sugar, cinnamon and nutmeg.

A further and more recently confirmed area of cinnamon's effectiveness is as an antiviral, especially in the mouth, for treating *E. coli* and candida. For people with type-2 diabetes cinnamon helps metabolise sugar, which means they can use it to reduce medication.

Cinnamon powder or tincture safely and gradually reduce cholesterol levels. Take a teaspoonful with each meal.

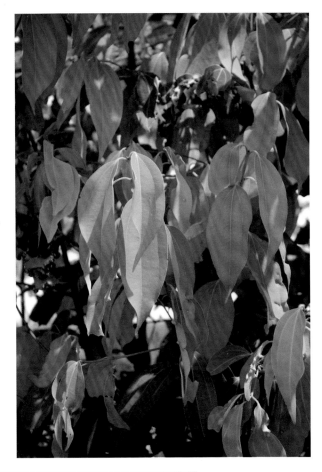

Cinnamon tincture
Fill a jar with **cinnamon sticks**. Pour on **vodka** to cover, and put away in a dark place for 3 or 4 weeks, shaking occasionally. Strain and bottle.

Dose: Take 1 teaspoonful 3 to 5 times a day for an infection, or 3 times a day for high cholesterol; 1 teaspoonful daily as a winter tonic.

Hot spiced apple juice
Put 2 litres of **apple juice** in a large saucepan. Add 2 sticks of **cinnamon**, and a tablespoon of **allspice** and a few **cloves**. You can also add a few slices of fresh **ginger** or a couple of **star anise**. Heat until just starting to boil, then turn the heat down low and let simmer until the flavours are well blended – about half an hour.

This is a deliciously warming winter drink, which can be enjoyed just for its taste, or it can be taken for colds and fevers.

Cinnamon tincture
- colds
- 'flu
- viral infections
- staph infections
- high cholesterol
- digestive problems

Hot spiced apple juice
- winter weather
- colds
- fevers

Caution: Cinnamon is a uterine stimulant so avoid large doses during pregnancy.

Cloves

Syzygium aromaticum, syn. *Eugenia aromatica, E. caryophyllata, E. caryophyllus*

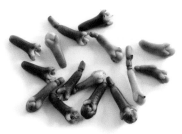

Cloves are the small flower buds of a large tropical tree, which as a desirable spice in trade has influenced the rise and fall of empires. It is best known, more modestly, as a toothache reliever, but also makes a powerful antiseptic and antispasmodic.

Myrtaceae
Myrtle family

Description: A tropical evergreen tree, to 12m (37ft), whose flower buds change from green to red, at which point they are picked; the unopened petals are the 'head' of the nail-like shape that gives the common name.

Distribution: Native to the Moluccas, Indonesia, now also grown in Zanzibar, Madagascar, other Indian Ocean islands and South Asia.

Related species: Many hundreds of other myrtle species, but cloves have had the most important role in history.

Parts used: Immature flower bud, dried; essential oil from bud, leaf and stem.

Above: fresh and dried cloves

It is somehow wonderful to know that a well-off Chinese, Indian or Egyptian of two, even three, thousand years ago would have done what you or I might do when we have a toothache: place a clove on the sore tooth or gum, and absorb its medicinal, numbing oil.

We now know about eugenol, the main active ingredient of clove, and its anaesthetic, antiseptic and antiviral action, but toothache needs quick relief, and that doesn't change over time.

An ancient use of cloves in China was for retainers approaching the emperor to chew a clove to prevent halitosis in the divine presence. It'll work for you when summoned to the big boss.

There's an interesting commonality in the name 'clove' itself. The scientific establishment now favours *Syzygium* over *Eugenia*, but the common name across cultures and over time has nearly always referenced the likeness of the fruit bud to an old round-headed nail, *clavus* in Latin, *clou* in French, *clove* in English.

What adds 'spice' to the clove story is that apart from the Arab, Indian and Chinese traders involved, for centuries nobody knew where cloves came from. There were rumours aplenty in Europe, where cloves were familiar to the Greeks and Romans and later in the Middle Ages, but the well-kept secret of clove's native terrain was kept until 1511.

It was then that state-sponsored Portuguese adventurers came across the remote Moluccas island group, athwart the Equator and near the Philippines, where the clove tree grew exclusively. This was officially Spanish territory so the Portuguese spice traders had to be careful, but with such a prize the truth soon came out.

There followed a fascinating and tangled story in which clove was both an object of trading desire while also the subject of official Church rejection.

Focusing on kitchen medicine, the best cloves are a rich brown colour with a full crown and plentiful oil. They are picked immature and dried as the distinctive flavour is lost when they ripen. Store them in glass and in the dark.

A tip for cooks when using cloves in, say, a bread sauce or a curry is to insert a few cloves into an onion, which is easily withdrawn when the flavour is sufficient. Much the same process goes into making a pomander to keep clothes fresh, when a fresh orange is studded with cloves and dried.

In addition to external medicinal uses, the oil of cloves goes into perfumes and pharmaceuticals, but is not a favoured massage oil since cloves can be an irritant to people with sensitive skins.

Somewhat ironically in terms of the ancient halitosis message, the main modern commercial use of cloves is to make cigarettes in Indonesia known as *kratek*. In India a clove serves to pin together the leaf used in the aromatic digestive mixture called *paan* or betel. It seems a strange fate for an ancient breath cleanser!

... as a flavouring [in cooking], cloves are best when kept below the level of recognition.
– Stobart (1980)

In view of their well-established reputation for this [toothache relief], it is strange that cloves are not more widely used on other parts of the body where they would be equally effective – for example, infused oil of cloves makes an excellent analgesic rub for backaches and headaches.
– Hedley & Shaw (1996)

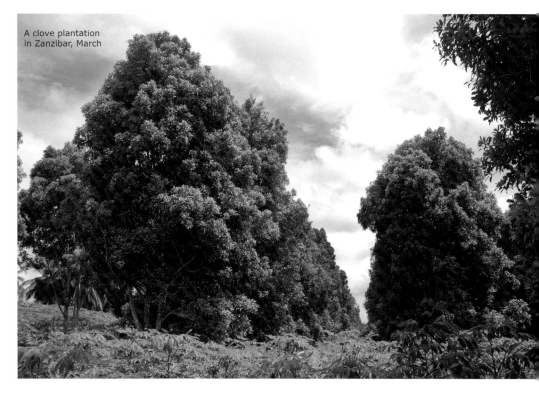

A clove plantation in Zanzibar, March

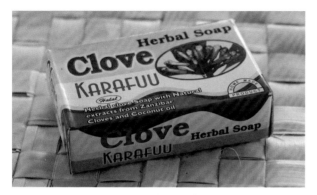

Caution: Do a 24 hour
skin patch test before
using cloves on your
skin as some people
are allergic. If you find
that either a clove or
the oil for toothache
irritates the inner
surfaces of the mouth,
discontinue use.

Do not use essential
oil of cloves during
pregnancy.

Clove & oat scrub
- jet lag
- tiredness
- hangovers
- use after massage
- clears the head

Use cloves for...

Cloves are a well-known warming stimulant, which works on a sluggish digestion and relieves indigestion. Internally, cloves taken as a tea or as clove water are an effective antispasmodic, ie allay nausea (taken with ginger), vomiting and excess flatulence.

In former times, along with other exotic aromatics, cloves were considered a plague or pestilence fighter. Today we know cloves make a good antiviral and disinfectant, which can help control candida and herpes.

Externally, cloves can be used as an antiseptic and analgesic lotion or scrub for massaging aches and joint pain, and the oil make a soothing compress for neuralgia.

Cloves have been found to be an effective blood thinner whose use can help prevent heart attacks and moderate altitude sickness.

Cloves are long established in Ayurveda for use during childbirth, where the stimulating effect assists in contractions. For this reason, using clove oil in pregnancy is contra-indicated.

Cloves are a traditional male aphrodisiac in the Middle and Far East, which may account both for its popularity and condemnation by religious authority.

As a final and less contested clove use, boiling up some cloves in hot water will make a suitably sweet but medicinal vapour in a sick room, which acts as a deodoriser and keeps mosquitoes away.

Clove and oat scrub

This recipe is our version of a traditional scrub used after massage on the island of Pemba in Zanzibar.

Put a handful of **cloves** in a bowl and pour on enough **boiling water** to cover them. Cover the bowl with a saucer and leave for about 15 minutes, then pour into a blender and mix until gritty. Add a handful of **rolled oats** and blend into a paste, adding more water if necessary.

Use straightaway, or keep in a jar in the fridge for a few days – the cloves preserve it naturally. Use as a scrub, leaving on for about ten minutes, then rinse off with warm water. It is wonderfully refreshing and invigorating, like instant air-conditioning in hot weather.

Coconut *Cocos nucifera*

Coconut is known in India as 'the tree that grants boons' and is arguably the most useful tree in the world. It is often the only cash crop on small tropical islands, supplies food and drink, shelter, wood for building, fuel, textile fibre, mats, thatching and basket materials, and has medicinal benefits.

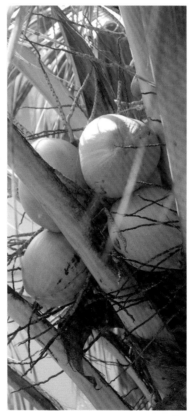

**Arecaceae
Palm family**

Description: A leaning palm, to 25m (80ft), with a tough single stem pitted with leaf scars (which provide a hold for climbing to harvest the fruit), pendulous fronds (to 8m or 25ft), small whitish flowers and large yellow–green fruits, in bunches of 10 to 20; each tree may yield 100–200 fruits a year.

Distribution: Maritime tropics worldwide, probably initially in SE Asia, but spread by traders and on ocean tides; commercially, both wild and in plantations.

Parts used: Locally practically everything on the tree has a value, but in kitchens the desiccated form of the copra or coconut milk/ cream and coconut oil are most likely to be kept.

Away from the tropics, the idea of coconut centres on the contents of the nut itself – its juice (coconut water) and flesh (copra) – rather than the manifold local economic uses of the whole fruit and the tree, with the odd coir welcome mat, made out of the fruit's fibres.

The raw juice is at first thin and bitter, and was once used as a purgative. Later it becomes creamy and jelly-like, sweeter and more nutritious. When you buy a coconut you need to hear the juice sloshing around, because this means the flesh will still be tasty and not dried out.

The flesh has some 50% water content; when it is dried to about 5% it is known as copra. Copra is stretched, grated and macerated into the dried form of commerce, desiccated coconut. It has the highest saturated fat content of any traded fat, but is low on protein and calorie counts.

There are two distinct liquid products: the original water or juice from the nut, and the 'milk' or 'cream' produced by grating the fresh nut or adding water to the desiccated copra. Coconut milk is

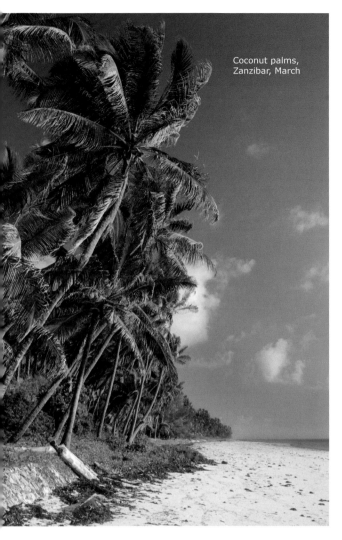
Coconut palms,
Zanzibar, March

In the West, the 'coconut cream' you purchase is a blend of the milk and cream, made from thin and thick squeezings of the 'milk' and 'cream' respectively.

Two older names of coconut, 'cocoanut' and 'cokernut', are seldom used these days.

Use coconut for...

There was a time when coconut was decried for its high saturated fat levels, which were thought to increase blood cholesterol levels and heart problems. More recently coconut has been claimed as having immune-protective qualities, which recommend it for use in treating 'flu, viral conditions and possibly HIV.

Perhaps both positions are being overstated, but there are well-recorded examples of other benefits. The milk is soothing and sustaining internally in cases of diarrhoea, Crohn's disease and irritable bowel, ulcerative colitis and mouth ulcers.

The oil is tolerated by people with steatorrhoea, a condition where normal fats are not absorbed. The oil is also a smooth, fragrant addition to skin ointments and massage creams, and as a hair conditioner. In Malaysia it was used as a haemorrhoid cream.

Taking extra virgin coconut oil internally for a month (dosage 3 tablespoons a day) has been found effective for treating ringworm

The coconut palm is one of Nature's greatest gifts to man. Nature gave it to him ready made, whereas whatever excellence is possessed by most of his other important food-plants has been his reward after ages of semi-conscious effort to ennoble them by selection.
– Burkhill (1935)

wonderful in cooking, with a rich taste, pure white hue and high fat content.

When making the milk or cream, at home or industrially, the oil rises and can be skimmed off. It has a low solidification point, at 30°C (85°F), and is used in cooking, in making margarine, soaps and beauty products, including shampoos.

and nail fungus. In India, fresh copra is a remedy for internal worms, including tapeworms.

Externally, oil rubbed into the scalp at bedtime on alternate days is an old headlice remedy; continue for at least 18 days, the incubation period of the lice eggs. Equal parts of coconut oil and bicarbonate of soda combine well in a home-made toothpaste; it will last a few days in the fridge.

Coconut in its various forms is a safe, non-toxic remedy, without side effects or harmful drug interactions.

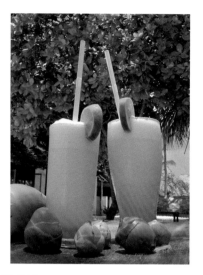

A cooling coconut milk and vanilla drink served with fresh limes: a welcome thirst-quencher at a beach resort in Zanzibar

Scalp conditioner
Melt ½ cup **coconut oil** in a small saucepan. Add 2 tablespoons crumbled dried **rosemary** (or chopped if fresh); infuse over a very low heat for half an hour. Strain and pour into a jar. To use, massage a little into the scalp – in a cold climate you will need to melt it in your hands first. After massaging, wrap your hair in a towel and leave for 15 or 20 minutes before shampooing as normal.

Coconut chutney
Put ½ cup **desiccated coconut** in a bowl and pour in ½ cup **boiling water**. Add 1 tablespoon **freshly grated ginger,** the juice of ¼ **lemon,** 1 teaspoonful **cumin powder** and **salt** to taste. Let it sit for about an hour, until the water is absorbed. An accompaniment to curries or other food.

Coconut anti-fungal ointment
Melt ½ cup of **coconut oil** in a small saucepan. Add 2 teaspoons **turmeric powder**. Take off the heat, pour into a jar and allow to cool.

Coconut milk
Combine equal parts **boiling water** and **desiccated coconut**, allow to sit for one hour, then squeeze through cheesecloth or a tea towel. Discard coconut pulp. Alternatively, bring to a boil one cup desiccated coconut plus one cup water, cool, mix in a blender at high speed, then strain and add water to the desired consistency.

Scalp conditioner
• dandruff
• itchy scalp
• thinning hair

Coconut chutney
• poor appetite
• weak digestion

Coconut anti-fungal ointment
• athlete's foot
• ringworm
• dandruff

Coffee _Coffea arabica, C. canephora_ (formerly _C. robusta_)

Rubiaceae
Madder family

Description: Small evergreen shrub growing to 5m (15ft) if left unpruned, normally kept at 2m (6ft); dark green leaves, fragrant white flowers and oval berries, ripening from green to yellow and red. Each berry has two seeds, which on picking are fermented, washed, dried and roasted, in roasts that vary from 'light' to 'very dark'.

Distribution: Indigenous to Ethiopia and Sudan, spreading with Arab empire, now pan-tropical. Brazil is the major producer.

Varieties: Some 90% of coffee trade is of the _arabica_ and _robusta_ varieties. This lack of genetic diversity may well be a critical issue.

Parts used: Bean, or seed, of coffee fruit.

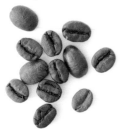

... a drink imitating that in the Stygian lake: black, thick and bitter.
– Sir Thomas Herbert, on first encountering coffee in Persia, 1620s

The 1650s were a caffeine age for London society, with the first tea, coffee and chocolate houses all opening, in spite of official, Cromwellian disapproval. Coffee's popularity has always gone hand in hand with religious or medical denunciation. While moderation may be boring it remains the best personal approach – meanwhile coffee's health profile is being reappraised, with many benefits accruing to its balance.

It is hard to imagine life without our familiar hot drinks, the legal and universal caffeine-rich staples of coffee, tea and chocolate. But Europe did not have cacao, the source of chocolate, before roughly 1528 (Spain), tea before 1610 (Holland) or coffee before 1615 (Venice) – though coffee did have a papal blessing (see below).

These bitter herbs combine well with sugar, which was newly available in trade, and with milk to make subtle, satisfying drinks that eventually became affordable to the common man.

But while still temperance drinks, these are also sensuous, democratic, addictive temptations, their very popularity a threat to secular and religious authority. As commodities they made fortunes for investors and governments, and offered a pretext for colonisation.

The church's ambivalence to coffee was cynically expressed by Pope Clement VIII (pope 1592–1605). Vatican officials were quick to denounce coffee as 'Satan's latest trap to catch Christian souls'. It was an Islamic plot, they charged, coffee being the drink of the Muslims, who were prohibited from wine, unlike good Christians.

Clement smelled the roasted beans, took a sip and pondered. He then decreed: 'This Satan's drink is so delicious that it would be a pity to let the infidels have exclusive use of it. We shall fool Satan by baptising it, and make it a truly Christian beverage.'

Coffee actually began as a sacrament, when in the thirteenth century Yemeni Sufis (dervishes) shared hot coffee communally before their ecstatic dances. This is the first record of the roasted beans, and coffee has been driving people wild ever since. It has now become the second most traded global commodity, after crude oil.

But it isn't just political or religious authority that will readily demonise and prohibit coffee: take medicine of our own day.

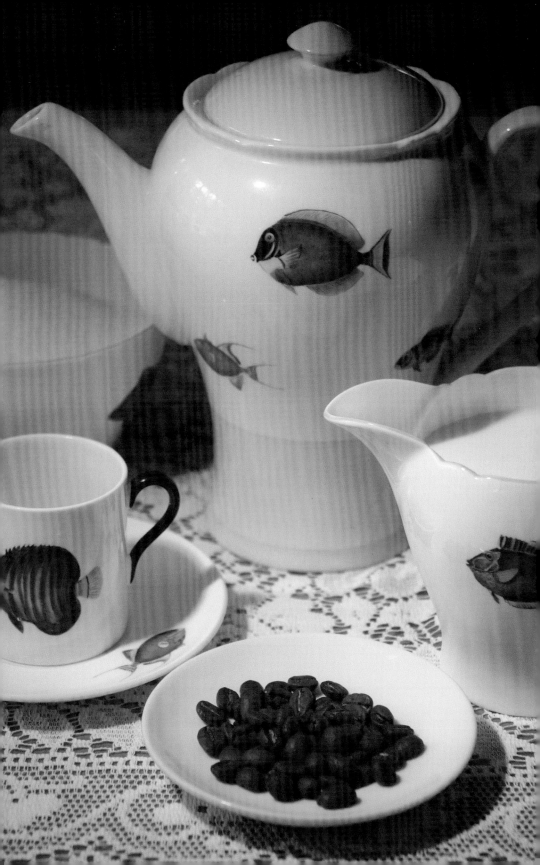

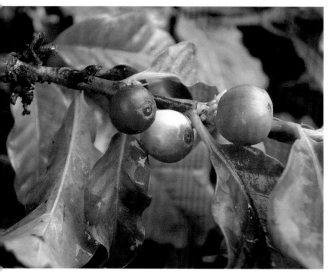

Ripening coffee beans, Kenya

Coffee helps digestion, and dispels wind: and it works gently by urine. The best way of taking it is as we commonly drink it, and there are constitutions for which it is very proper.
– Hill (1812)

[Coffee is the] *only herbal remedy shown consistently to extend life in epidemiological studies.*
– Bergner (2009)

Caution: Coffee should be avoided if you suffer from palpitations, hyperactivity, anxiety or insomnia.

Go to your health practitioner, and it is quite likely that you will be told to stop coffee. But, as American herbalist Paul Bergner explains, coffee is now a high source of dietary antioxidants in the average North American diet. While coffee has less antioxidants than some fruits (eg blackberries and cranberries) or a vegetable like artichoke, it is taken in more volume and more habitually than these foods. Bergner warns: 'This may be a critical consideration before recommending that individuals remove coffee from their diets.' Coffee is also one of the few bitters we consume.

Bergner performs the useful service of showing that many of the reasons why coffee is a 'bad' thing have been challenged in recent focused research, as we will see.

Use coffee for...

Moderation is the key to coffee. Bergner cites up to six cups a day as moderate usage; it has been estimated, by the way, that a lethal dose is 66 cups of 5oz (140g) size.

A huge Harvard research study, with 120,000 people participating, demonstrated that two to four cups of coffee for women and four to six cups for men were beneficial for mortality, mainly because of a reduction in cardiac death. Coffee is developing a well-attested influence on increasing human longevity, but with higher intake the effect turned negative.

In terms of cardiovascular disease, coffee elevates blood pressure only to a minor degree, research shows, and most kinds of blood cholesterol hardly at all. Filtering coffee appears to remove the constituents that raise lipid levels.

Coffee taken in moderation seems to protect sufferers of type-2 diabetes, probably through its active antioxidant content.

Meta-analysis demonstrates a research consensus that coffee is protective against liver cancer, but is neutral for breast, colon, thyroid and pancreatic cancer. Bladder cancer may be linked to coffee drinking, though analysis shows this finding was not controlled for nicotine. This means that smokers who also drink coffee may be at greater risk because of their smoking.

Coffee is mildly diuretic and laxative, and aids in digestion either before or after meals, as we know by experience. Less familiar is that moderate coffee intake is protective for gastrointestinal and gallbladder problems, Parkinson's disease and Alzheimer's disease.

What, then, of the charges that coffee increases levels of insomnia, anxiety and depression and causes difficulties in pregnancy? Sleep is jokingly said to be a symptom of coffee deprivation, but it is a real issue for occasional users or those who exceed their normal intake. Moderation and commonsense are again called for, as far as possible.

Anxiety, tachycardia, premenstrual stress and most kinds of clinical depression are dose-dependent in relation to coffee; high dosage will exacerbate embedded symptoms, as will smoking. The linking of coffee, particularly caffeine, to problems in pregnancy is controversial. Evidence that caffeine builds up in the foetus and takes longer to be excreted is worrying, as is a possible connection to foetal growth restriction and increased risk of miscarriage. If in doubt, it is best to avoid coffee in pregnancy.

But charges that coffee raises risk of osteoporosis or has negative effects on the adrenals have been robustly questioned. These and older 'certainties' are being rescrutinised (and not just by coffee industry funding), and coffee's balance sheet is being redrawn.

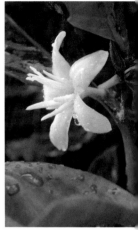

The exquisite flower of coffee, Kenya, March

Coffee: constitutional right, if right for your constitution

For making coffee at home, we prefer freshly ground beans, using about a tablespoonful per person. We grind these in an electric grinder, along with a few pods of cardamom, then filter in a cafetière. The cardamom takes the edge off the jitteriness coffee can cause but without diminishing its stimulant effect. Other spices we often grind in are some combination of licorice and vanilla, cola nut or chocolate.

The finer you grind the beans the stronger and more bitter the result; and the longer you brew your coffee the bitterer and more astringent it will be. We find one cup a morning of such a brew entirely satisfying.

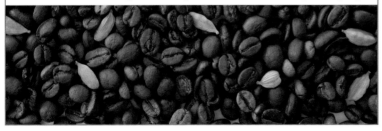

Once roasted, ground and infused, myriad different aromatic molecules combine with protein, oil, tannins, sugar, starch, fibre, caffeine and bitter phenolic substances to imbue coffee with a wonderfully complex taste.
– Kapoor (2003)

It can scarcely be doubted that tea and coffee would have been much more employed therapeutically had their habitual use as articles of diet not limited their application.
– Bentley & Trimen (1880)

Coriander, cilantro *Coriandrum sativum*

**Apiaceae
(Umbelliferae)
Carrot family**

Description: Small hardy annual or perennial, up to 50cm (20in) high, with finely cut top leaves and broader lower leaves, small, flat umbels of white–pink flowers, followed by round green fruits ripening to brown; plants have a characteristic leaf smell before becoming aromatic and spicy in the fruit.

Distribution: Native to Mediterranean basin and southern Europe, spreading across hot temperate zones into Asia and introduced first into South and Central America, later North America.

Other corianders: Unrelated but bearing the name coriander are false coriander (*Eryngium foetidum*); Roman coriander (*Nigella sativa*) and Vietnamese coriander (*Polygonum odoratum*).

Parts used: Lower leaves (which resemble parsley) and upper leaves (which resemble dill or carrot); fruit (incorrectly called seed); essential oil.

Like dill, its cousin, coriander is an ancient herb grown domestically and commercially for its green leaf and later its fruit or seeds, equivalent to two bites at the culinary and medicinal cherry. Both plants are excellent digestive remedies, but coriander has a further claim: its leaves have acquired their own name, cilantro, and a 'love it or hate it' reputation.

Archaeological records show that coriander was used in the Middle East some 7,000 years ago, and it spread from its ancestral home around the Old World, and thence to North and Central America.

Remains of coriander fruit have been found in the tomb of Ramses II, and it was both food and medicine in ancient Egypt, India and China. Its early domestication is recognised in the choice of 'sativum' ('cultivated') in its name.

There are Old Testament references to coriander: in both Exodus and Numbers it is compared to manna, which is said to be 'white like coriander'; it may be the herb's digestive effect that was valued in this phrase.

The Romans are thought to have brought coriander to Britain, and it was commercially grown until recent times. It needs a hot summer to ripen the fruit but for most everyday users having the

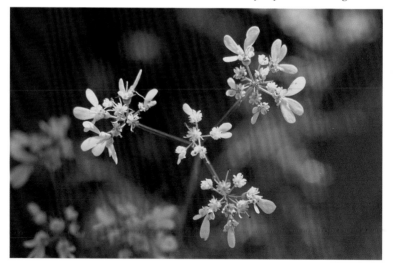

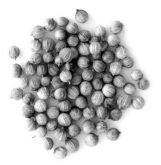

leaves to hand in a pot or in the garden is enough.

Coriander fruit flavoured the medieval wine and spice mixture known as hippocras, and was used to make confits or digestive sweets until Edwardian times. In 1609 Sir Hugh Plat wrote in his book *Delights for Ladies*: 'A quarter pound of coriander seeds and three pounds of sugar will make great, huge and big comfrets.'

In Chinese tradition, coriander also had 'delights' as a herb of immortality and as an aphrodisiac. It certainly had an aphrodisiac reputation in the Middle East, and there are plentiful such references to it in *Tales of the Arabian Nights*.

But there was always a fuss about the smell of the leaves. The Roman naturalist Pliny (AD 23–79) is said to have named coriander after the Greek *koris*, for stink bug, both having the same bad smell.

The old English herbals are full of complaints of the awfulness of the green phase of coriander's growth (see Parkinson alongside).

We find the fuss overblown and delight in the fresh and lively aroma of growing coriander tops. These take the name *cilantro* (from the Spanish) or Chinese parsley in North America, and *dhania* in India; one author calls coriander leaves 'the most commonly used garnish in India'.

In our own kitchen we add fresh coriander leaves to curries and naan bread, or sprinkle them on soups and fresh salads. Millions of cooks around the world agree, whether they are using coriander in stir-fries or salsas, boerewors or sambhar, a tea or a chutney.

Perhaps people are genetically predisposed either to like or hate coriander leaf. The naysayers talk of a rank or soapy smell that they instinctively dislike. To judge by the way fresh coriander or cilantro is found in supermarkets these days, and not just in ethnic stores, it is now mainstream.

The seed also has commercial uses based on its flavour. In London's nineteenth-century gin palaces coriander was a cheaper option to juniper, and it is still added to some gins, to tobacco, chewing gum and perfumes.

A former herbal use of the strong taste of coriander was to mask that of domestic purgatives such as rhubarb or senna. And to cap the irony of the bad smell coming good, coriander has a reputation in China as a breath freshener.

The fresh leaf is probably the most widely used of all flavouring herbs throughout the world.
– Stuart (1979)

... the whole plant, seede and all while it is greene and growing hath a strong and loathsome savour scarce to be endured, but when the seede is full ripe and dry it is of a reasonable good sent and taste without offence.
– Parkinson (1640)

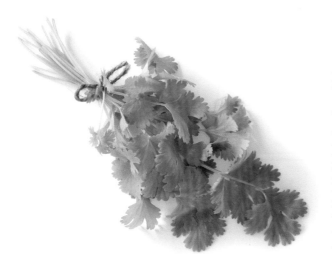

juice contains plentiful iron and vitamins A, B and C.

Building on this eliminative quality, in Ayurveda, the traditional holistic system of Indian medicine, coriander tea has a role in the safe excretion of heavy metals like lead, arsenic or mercury. Sebastian Pole explains that this is done carefully through drop doses with a toxin absorption agent like chlorella.

The tea is also used in Ayurveda for treating kidney problems, with the fruit boiled in water as a decoction. The same remedy is applied in India as an eyewash.

Used externally, a damp poultice made from coriander fruit crushed in a pestle and mortar or powdered in your coffee grinder can be applied to rheumatic joints to ease the pain. This worked in ancient Egypt and should be effective for you today. Add a little hot water to the crushed seeds, and you can use cornmeal or flour to thicken the paste.

Note, though, that some people may find the oils in coriander irritating on the skin, so if you develop rashes or red blotches, be ready to abandon this treatment.

Overall coriander has a reputation as a safe remedy, without counter-indications or drug interactions. It is certainly not the monster of foul smell and bad repute that many people have depicted.

[Coriander] comforts a cold and moist Stomach, helps Digestion, stops Vomiting, kills Worms, and stops all fluxes: after Meat it closes the Mouth of the Stomach, and suppresses Vapours that would hurt the head.
– Salmon (1696)

The flower water is a fantastic antispasmodic.
– Pole (2008)

Use coriander for...

Medicinally both leaves and fruit of coriander are rich in volatile oils that act beneficially on the digestive system. The appetite is stimulated, and in India coriander is used to interest anorexic patients in food. In Parkinson's words, the fruit 'is very comfortable to the stomacke'.

Moreover, as he says, it 'resisteth forcible paines of the winde chollicke'; in our terms, coriander is a carminative, a herb that eases flatulence, indigestion and gas.

Whether the fruits are taken as a tea or by chewing, coriander is antispasmodic, meaning it helps settle spasms and cramp in the gut, and associated tension headaches.

A juice made from grinding the leaves has an expectorant property, and will help release mucus from the lungs by stimulating the cough reflex. The

Coriander tea

Coriander seed should have a fresh lemony taste. To extract the most flavour, crush the seed before making the tea. Use 1 tablespoon crushed **coriander seed** to 2 or 3 cups **boiling water**. Brew for 5 minutes.

Dukka

This delicious recipe is a traditional Egyptian seasoning. Traditionally eaten at breakfast, as a dry dip for warm flatbread dipped first in olive oil, dukka can be used as a seasoning for beans, humous, salads – use your imagination.

Roast ½ cup (50g) **hazelnuts** in a medium oven for about 10 minutes. Rub off the skins. Use a dry frying pan on moderate heat to toast ½ cup (75g) **sesame seeds**, then ½ cup (30g) **coriander seed** and ¼ cup (15g) **cumin seed**. Grind all ingredients in a mortar or on pulse in a blender until coarsely ground – don't grind too finely or it may go oily. Add **salt** to taste. Stored in an airtight container, it will keep for several months.

Hippocras

This spiced wine was very popular in the Middle Ages, and there are many different recipes. We've made our version with white wine as it goes well with the lemony taste of the coriander.

Put 500ml (1 pint or 2 cups) **white wine** in a saucepan. Add 1 tablespoon crushed **coriander seed**, 1 or 2 slices **fresh ginger** and a few **peppercorns**. Heat gently for half an hour but do not allow it to boil.

Add 2 teaspoons of **honey**, or to taste and pour (unstrained) into a bottle or large jar. Leave to infuse for a few days, then strain and bottle.

Cilantro and lemon lotion/sauce

Blend the **juice of 2 lemons** with an equal amount of **olive oil** until emulsified and creamy. Add a handful or two of **fresh coriander leaves** and blend until smooth.

Use fresh or store in the fridge for several days until needed. Use as a face, hand and body lotion, or drizzle on vegetables or pasta – after all, folk wisdom says 'don't put anything on your skin that you can't eat'.

Coriander tea
- irritable bowel
- tension headache
- kidney problems

Dukka
- digestion
- appetite

Hippocras
- appetite
- digestion
- colds and chills
- circulation

Cilantro & lemon lotion
- dry skin
- freckles
- chapped hands

Corn, maize *Zea mays*

**Graminae (Poaceae)
Grass family**

Description: Tall,
sturdy annual, to 4m
(12ft); stalks bear male
flowers at the top (the
beard or tassels)
and female flowers
part-way up, in leaf
joints (the cob or
ears). Rows of close-
packed milky seeds,
with threads (silk),
10–20cm (4–8in) long
and protective opaque
leaves (husks).

Distribution:
Indigenous to Central
and northern South
America; now grown
worldwide in temperate
and subtropical areas.

Related species: Not
closely related to other
grasses.

Parts used: Silky
threads, dried for a
pleasant tea; cornflour
(cornstarch).

Corn, maize, Indian corn or sweetcorn has become the leading global cereal crop, and supplies food for humans and animals, corn oil, syrup and starch, breakfast cereal, popcorn and bourbon whisky. It is also an estimable herbal remedy, with cornsilk from the cob being dried to make a tea for urinary tract complaints and cornflour a substitute for talcum powder.

Corn may not be the tallest commercial grass (this honour goes to sugar cane), but it is the most widespread. Crop projections for 2019 put global corn output at 1083 million tonnes, against wheat at 757mt and rice 516mt. Corn also had the highest rate of tonnage increase, having overtaken wheat and rice in the early 2000s.

In much of the Americas, across sub-Saharan Africa, parts of Europe, Asia and Australia corn is the staple crop for humans and animals alike. New early ripening cultivars now enable it to mature at the limits of its growing range, in Scotland, for example.

It is a long-held argument that growing cereals enabled the spread of human culture and growth of cities. Early great civilisations in Mesopotamia, China, Egypt, and India had reliable supplies, and the conquering Spanish found the same thing in Mexico and northern South America in the

early sixteenth century. Corn was grown alongside beans and squash, the 'three sisters', and was the basis of thriving cultures from Argentina to Canada. It was a perfect combination, the beans climbing up the corn, and feeding nitrogen into the roots, and the squash leaves protecting the soil and shading out weeds. Moreover – and a fact not understood by the conquerors and settlers – the three crops together made up for nutritional deficiencies in the corn.

Over thousands of years of corn cultivation the native Americans learned that it needed to be soaked overnight in water with lime or wood ash before being ground into meal. It was only in the 1930s that this process, nixtamalisation, was finally explained by scientists.

Corn contains vitamin B3, niacin, but this is locked in until released by an alkali such as lime or ash. B3 deficiency from monoculture of corn can lead to pellagra, a scourge of southern Europe and

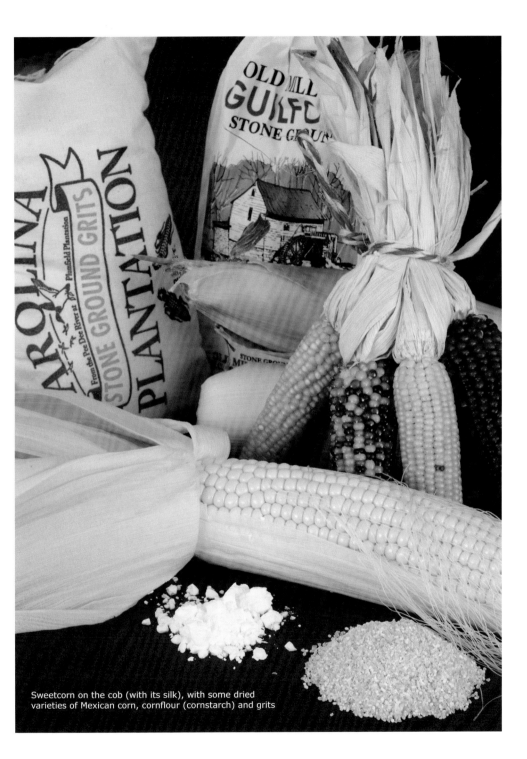

Sweetcorn on the cob (with its silk), with some dried
varieties of Mexican corn, cornflour (cornstarch) and grits

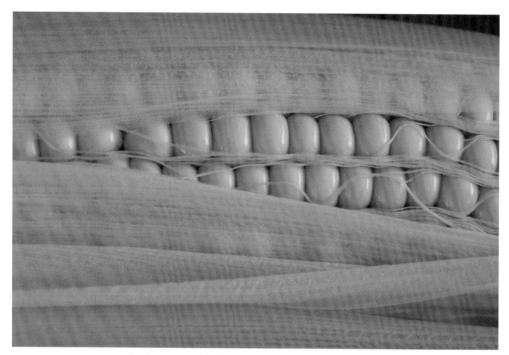

the American South in the nine-teenth and early twentieth cen-turies. In the first ten months of 1915, 1,300 people succumbed to pellagra in South Carolina alone.

This affliction, typified by '4Ds' – diarrhoea, dermatitis, dementia and death – was remedied by processing the corn as native Americans did. Facing climate change, we could learn from them again by adopting a 'three sisters' method of crop combining.

Use corn/maize for...

It is a strange thing that the most medicinal part of corn is always thrown away before cooking the cob. It may be surprising that cornsilk, the fine threads that are attached to the cob, shown above with the husk leaves, is an 'official' diuretic and urinary demulcent in the *British Herbal Pharmacopoeia*.

What this means is that taking a tea made with fresh or dried cornsilk assists the body to produce urine and is soothing to the urinary tract. Conditions such as cystitis, urethritis and prostatitis, along with oedema (water retention) and kidney dysfunction are all benefited by the gentle effects of cornsilk tea.

This has been called one of the best natural diuretics, especially as it combines this quality with a soothing action on the kidneys and bladder. It is a front-line remedy, for the first signs of urinary unease, when early action can flush away the infection. It is antiseptic, restorative and pain-relieving. Oddly for a diuretic, in small doses it can alleviate bedwetting.

Other symptoms you can help relieve by cornsilk tea include high blood pressure and fluid retention.

In China cornsilk is known as 'jade rice whiskers' and is used for treatment of kidney stone, but this is not a home remedy: consult your doctor or herbalist.

Cornsilk tea is safe, pleasant and has no side effects or contra-indications; it is also supplied free with your cob!

Cornflour is processed to remove the protein and leave only corn starch. This is used commercially in talcum-free body powders. It makes an excellent baby powder just as it is, to keep babies' bottoms dry and comfortable, and prevent nappy rash.

Julie uses cornflour combined with turmeric for fungal infections, and adding bicarbonate of soda (as in the recipe below) keeps feet smelling fresh.

Tropical talcum powder.
– Duke (1997)

Midwestern manna.
– Gill (2007)

Cornsilk tea
Buy fresh, milky cobs. Gather the silk, to use fresh or dry it for later use by spreading it on brown paper to dry. (Meanwhile, boil the cobs in salted water and enjoy with lashings of butter.)

Use about a tablespoonful of fresh **cornsilk** or a teaspoonful of the chopped, dried cornsilk and infuse in a cup of **boiling water**. Leave to brew for at least five minutes. Take either hot or cold, up to three times a day.

Scented body powder
Mix a cup of **cornflour** with a few drops of your favourite **essential oil**, stirring in well. Lavender and rose are often used.

Rub through a sieve to get it smooth again, then keep in a jar and use as needed to keep skin dry and comfortable.

Foot powder
Sieve 1 cup **cornflour**, half a cup of **turmeric powder** and half a cup of **bicarbonate of soda**, or equivalent proportions.

Store in a jar and use a small amount daily to keep feet free from smells and fungal infections.

Cornsilk tea
- cystitis
- bladder irritation
- urethritis
- prostatitis
- fluid retention

Scented body powder
- heat rash
- dampness
- fungal infections

Foot powder
- athlete's foot
- smelly feet

Cranberry *Vaccinium macrocarpon*

**Ericaceae
Heather family**

Description: Low-growing (to 50cm, 20in) matted, creeping perennial, tangled with moss and grass in peat bogs; small, leathery green leaves; flowers whitish-pink; berries, green at first and bright red when mature.

Distribution: Wild and commercially grown in northern areas of USA and Canada, Europe and Great Britain, in bogs, swamps and areas of acid soils.

Related species: Small cranberry (*V. oxycoccos*), mountain cranberry or ligonberry (*V. vitis-idaea*); bilberries and blueberries are closely related *Vacciniums*.

Parts used: Berries and their juice; also capsules of concentrated juice.

Like puppies, cranberries are not just for Christmas! Best known as a sweetened sauce accompanying turkey at Christmas and Thanksgiving Day, these sharp and sour deep red fruits have all-year medicinal benefits, in berry, juice and other forms.

The name 'cranberry' is obscure, though a plausible suggestion is that the early American colonists thought the folded-back flowers and long single stamen resembled the neck of a crane and called the plant a 'crane-berry'.

Certainly the Pilgrim Fathers arriving in North America in 1620 would have delighted in a native cranberry twice the size of its European cousins and equally good to use. It combined well with local turkey meat and it was soon a staple of Thanksgiving feasts as a sauce, cooked with apples and honey to reduce its sharpness.

Not only was cranberry sauce pleasingly piquant, the berries also kept for months without extra treatment. Containing benzoic acid, a natural preservative, they were stored in American kitchens and cellars through harsh winters, and also exported to Europe. The old method for choosing berries to undertake the Atlantic voyage was to tip them down a flight of stairs. Good berries bounced to the bottom while unsound ones stayed on the steps. The same principle is reproduced in modern US cranberry-sorting machines.

Use cranberries for...

The bulk of the cranberry consumption today is as juice, in both sweetened and unsweetened formats. The unsweetened is preferable for its better immune-supporting qualities and if you are calorie-counting.

Cranberries have a high vitamin C content and tannins that make them astringent, but crucially they also contain arbutin. This chemical compound is antibiotic and diuretic, with a special capacity to block *E. coli* in the urinary tract. It appears to cause a 'receptor blockade' in the bladder walls, so that harmful bacteria like *E. coli* are denied a foothold and are flushed harmlessly in the urine.

This rare property underlies why cranberry juice is a classic treatment for cystitis, a very painful consequence of *E. coli* infecting the bladder. Two glasses of cranberry juice a day (about half a litre) are a sufficient adult dose to stop cystitis taking hold in a high-risk individual. In acute cases where infection is present, the dosage might be doubled for a few days. With all urinary tract infections care should be taken

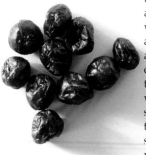

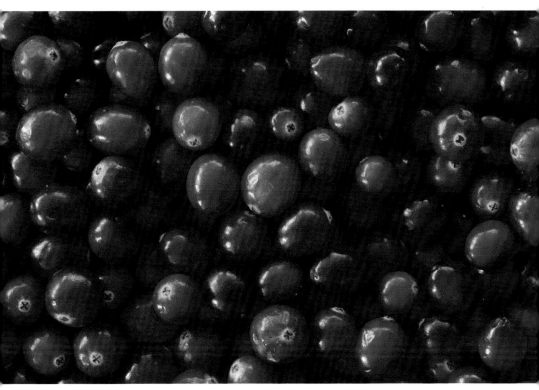

– see your doctor immediately if you suspect the infection may be affecting your kidneys, in which case antibiotics are needed.

Laboratory trials suggest that cranberry juice will similarly block the harmful bacteria *Heliobacter pylori*, which can cause ulcers in the stomach, and be effective against salmonella poisoning. Cranberry may help reduce prostate symptoms. If its antioxidants, as has been proposed, can stop platelets in the blood gluing together, this would make blood clots less likely and hence prevent heart attack and stroke. Cranberry has also been used to reduce diarrhoea and nausea, and is well tolerated by people with diabetes mellitus.

A well-known household remedy, cranberry is commonly taken for urinary tract problems such as cystitis and urethritis. Sharp-flavoured and rich in vitamin C, it has strong disinfectant properties within the urinary and gastrointestinal tracts. – Chevallier (2007)

Cranberry and raspberry shortbread

Instead of drinking cranberry juice all the time, which is hard work, try this shortbread. The raspberry and sugar sweeten the taste just enough.

Cream 1 cup (250g) **butter** and ½ cup **brown sugar** until fluffy. Mix in 2½ cups **flour** to make a crumbly dough. Add ½ cup dried **cranberries** and ¼ cup **raspberries** (fresh or unfrozen). Mix again, spread into a flat, greased pan. Bake at 300°F (160°C) for half an hour. Cool and cut into squares.

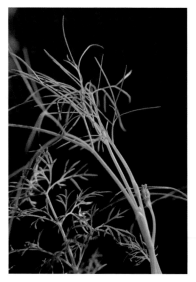

Cumin *Cuminum cyminum*

**Apiaceae
(Umbelliferae)
Carrot family**

Description: Slender, small annual, growing to 30cm (12in); bears tall, sparse umbels of pinky-white flowers and small, beige, bristly ridged fruit.

Distribution: Indigenous to the upper Nile and Mediterranean generally, cultivated in North Africa, Middle East, India and China.

Related species: Caraway (*Carum carvi*). Black cumin (*Nigella sativa*) is not related; confusingly, this plant is also known as nutmeg flower and Roman coriander.

Parts used: Dried ripe fruit (seeds), essential oil.

When one is tired of all seasonings, cumin remains welcome.
– Pliny (1st century AD)

They [seeds] are of a very disagreeable flavour, but of excellent virtues.
– Hill (1812)

... a superb addition to any formula where there is a compromised digestive system.
– Pole (2006)

Cumin in your kitchen is often used for making Indian food, and you might suppose it is a spice of Indian origin. Actually native to Egypt, it was once grown widely in Europe as a condiment and used medicinally for digestive problems, coughs and chest conditions, and insomnia.

An Old World spice of the Egyptians and mentioned in the Old Testament, cumin was loved by the Romans, who used it much as we now use pepper, as a table condiment, with bread and wine.

It remained popular in Europe during the monastic period as a medicinal spice and was widely grown in the British Isles, only to be replaced by the stronger-smelling caraway in the last three hundred years or so.

Cumin continued to be grown in Britain, and as recently as the coronation of George VI, in 1937, a Cornish farmer presented the king with a pound of his special cumin.

Whether the king liked the smell is not recorded, but some people cannot stand it. In Indian cuisine, the pungency is valued, and most curries begin with the sound of cumin seeds (*jeera*) popping in hot oil before other spices are added.

At home we regularly use cumin when cooking beans, as they do in Mexico. It is also integral to couscous in North Africa, kebabs in the Middle East, stews in Spain and pies in the US.

Cumin is used as a pickling spice, in flavouring several Dutch and German cheeses, and is added to some breads and cakes. Commercially it goes into a distilled essential oil, liqueurs and perfume. Veterinarians use cumin in treating digestive problems of animals and birds.

Use cumin for…

In herbalists' terms, cumin is a carminative, which means it works on the digestive system to relieve gas, bloating and griping pains as well as to promote digestion generally. Sebastian Pole's textbook on Ayurveda states that cumin is 'one of the best herbs for digestive sluggishness'.

It is no accident that our modern kitchen cupboards hold various other spices kept for much the same carminative purpose, such as anise, caraway, fennel, dill and ginger.

Cumin's pungency being of a drying nature, its particular value is in stimulating slow or 'damp' digestions all the way through the system, from freshening the breath to easing diarrhoea.

Cumin has an old reputation in relieving coughs, by relaxing a tight chest and helping move mucus out. For extra stimulation combine with ginger and pepper, as a tea or a flavoured water. As with other aromatics, dry-roasting the seeds slightly before use brings out maximum flavour.

Another former use for cumin was as a relieving eye compress made from the tea. Edmund Spenser in 1590 described

The wholesome saulge [sage]*, and lavender still gray, / Ranke-smelling rue, and cummin good for the eyes.*

Cousin caraway

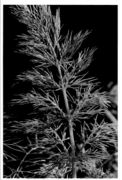

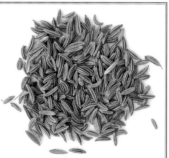

Caraway (*Carum carvi*) is another aromatic umbellifer with a North African and Mediterranean origin. A biennial, it is similar in appearance to cumin in both foliage and fruits, as the illustrations show; it has similar culinary and medicinal uses, although it is closer to dill seed in taste. Mrs Grieve (1931) relates how caraway's 'former extensive employment in medicine has much decreased in recent years'. It is perhaps best known today for its slightly bitter, mild and nutty flavour, used in rye bread, liqueurs and seedy cake. Herbally, it is a carminative, taken to relieve indigestion and colic, and has been used for children with stomach or respiratory problems, though not all can tolerate the taste.

Where poor digestion or persistent cough lead to headache, cumin tea offers some prospect of relief. For headache linked to insomnia, an Ayurvedic recipe suggests a teaspoon of fried cumin seeds with a ripe banana before bed.

Like fennel, cumin is used in India to increase breast milk production, and stimulate slow menstruation. These qualities suggest it is wise to avoid using cumin in pregnancy.

The oil is extracted by distillation and used in perfumery and in liqueurs such as the German kümmel. Cumin is also used in veterinary medicine.

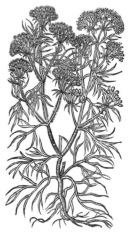

Cumin, from Parkinson's *Theatrum Botanicum* (1640)

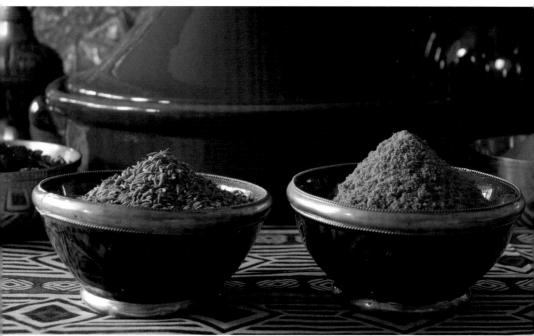

Whole and ground
seeds of cumin

Cumin tea
- gas & flatulence
- weak digestion
- coughs

Digestive tea
- colic
- griping pains
- abdominal gas
- flatulence
- indigestion
- nausea
- over-eating

Jaljeera
- dehydration
- hot weather

Cumin tea
Use about ½ teaspoonful of **cumin seeds** per cup of **boiling water**, and infuse for about 5 minutes. Drink after meals or as needed.

Digestive tea
Mix together roughly equal amounts of dried **cumin seed**, **coriander seed**, **fennel seed** (or aniseed), **fenugreek seed** and twice the amount of **peppermint**.

Use about a teaspoonful of the mixture per cup of **boiling water**, and infuse, covered, for about 5 minutes. Strain and drink hot or cool.

Cumin salt
Mix a few **cumin seeds** with **coarse salt crystals** and put in a salt mill. Grind as needed for use.

Jaljeera
This is a refreshing and thirst-quenching drink from India.

Grind with a mortar and pestle: 2 tablespoons **cumin** (dry roasted), 3 tablespoons chopped fresh **mint** leaves and 1 or 2 tablespoons chopped **coriander leaves**. Mix with 4 tablespoons **tamarind purée** (or **lemon juice**), 1 tablespoon **brown sugar** (or to taste), a pinch or two of **salt**, ½ teaspoon **chilli powder** (optional). Add 5 cups **water**, garnish with mint leaves and serve with or without ice.

Dill

Anethum graveolens, A. sowa

**Apiaceae
(Umbelliferae)
Carrot family**

Description:
Aromatic annual
umbellifer that reaches
75cm (30in), with
hollow stems, feather-
like leaves (known as
dill weed) and small
yellow flowers, followed
by flat, light brown fruit
(dill seeds).

Distribution: Native to
Mediterranean, central
and south Asia, and
widely cultivated in
temperate Europe and
USA.

Related species:
Caraway seed (*Carum
carvi*) is probably the
closest in flavour to dill
seed, and can be used
as a substitute.

Parts used: Leaves,
dried ripe fruit (seeds),
essential oil.

*This is the herb of
choice for children's
colic.*
– Hoffmann (2003)

*On a hot day in
Virginia, I know nothing
more comforting than a
fine spiced* [dill] *pickle,
brought up trout-like,
from the sparkling
depths of the aromatic
jar below the stairs of
Aunt Sally's cellar.*
*– Thomas Jefferson
(late eighteenth
century)*

**Dill seed is renowned as the first-choice
soothing, safe treatment for babies
with colic, in the form of gripe water.
It also works well to settle adult stomachs
suffering from acid indigestion, gas and the
like; it can be safely recommended to nursing
mothers.**

Dill is an ancient herb, with
millennia-old recorded histories
in Egypt and India. It came to
western Europe with the Roman
empire, and travelled to North
America with the Puritans. It
acquired the name 'meetin' seed'
there from its use as a children's
chew during long hours in chapel.

The name 'dill' is variously
claimed as originating in Anglo-
Saxon or Old Norse, but in either
case its meaning was 'to lull or
soothe', from the plant's primary
use in calming upset infants.

Like its umbelliferous relative,
coriander, dill is two herbs in
one, the leaves and the seeds
enabling both an earlier and a later
tasting of the plant's culinary and
medicinal virtues.

In dill's case the dark green
feathery foliage of summer (dill
weed) is followed in the autumn
by the fruit (dill seed), which is
beige in colour, thin, light and
semi-transparent. The leaves
tend to be used more in cooking

for sauces and to give a tang to
cabbage and potatoes (and curries
in India), as well as yogurt.

The flowers and top leaves flavour
the cucumbers in dill pickle, along
with garlic and salt; it is estimated
by Pickle Packers International
that every American consumes 100
individual dill pickles (or 9lb of
the stuff) a year.

The dried fruits of dill (not
actually seeds) are generally the
herbal component and the flavour
is more concentrated in them. The
first taste on chewing is savoury,
followed by a slight bitterness and
after that a pungent aftertaste.
There is no sweetness, but the
effect is satisfying and the breath
feels cleaned and the saliva is
stimulated.

Use dill for…

Gripe water is the commercial
form of the dill tea we describe
in our recipe. Some contributors
to an American online herbal
forum complained not long ago
that their purchased gripe water

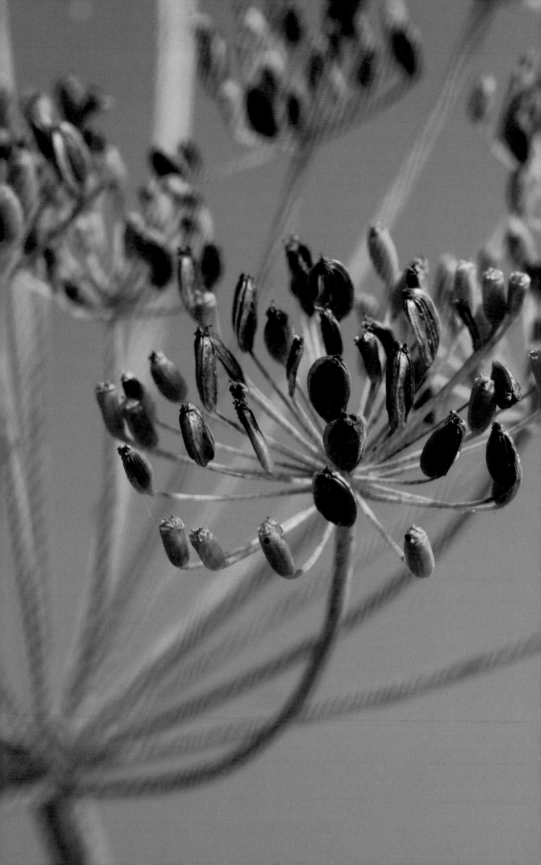

was expensive and moreover was high in alcohol. How this could be thought to be good for babies is a moot point, but a home-made dill tea is cheap, appropriate and beneficial.

Dill has a long tradition as a strong emmenagogue, meaning it works to assist menstruation, taken in the form of a tea. For this reason pregnant women are advised not to take dill in medicinal concentrations, though, as ethnobotanist Jim Duke said, this does not mean dill pickles are banned if you are pregnant!

There is another caution for people who handle fresh dill in large quantities, such as herbal farm workers. The active ingredient in dill, carvone, can cause blistering or burning of the skin on prolonged contact and can also reduce the skin's natural protection in bright sunlight.

But all other groups in the population can rely on dill as safe and reliable to use. The vigour of carvone is the means by which dill freshens the breath, stops hiccups, soothes the discomfort of heartburn. Technically, it is known as a carminative.

It is a good antiseptic; it also kills insects. Dill is a sedative herb, and a cup of dill tea taken before bedtime should help you achieve restful sleep. Rich in minerals, it is also good in salt-free diets.

It [dill] is also put among pickled Cowcumbers, wherewith it doth very well agree, giving unto the cold fruit a pretty spicie taste or rellish. It being stronger than Fenell, is of the more force to expell winde in the body. Some use to eate the seed to stay Hickocke [hiccups].
– Parkinson (1629)

Dill tea (gripe water)

The Rolls-Royce of gripe waters is organic dill aromatic water distilled by Welsh herbal company Avicenna, which is to dill tea as a 12-year-old single malt is to blended whisky, but a home-made tea is still a good starting point.

Crush 1 teaspoon **dill seeds** in a mortar and boil with a **cup of water** for at least 5 minutes or until the liquid is reduced by a half. Allow to cool to room temperature, and give to your infant in a baby bottle or via a small spoon. Keep for one day only and then make more.

Alternatively, crush and boil similar amounts of anise and caraway, alone or all three together, finding by experimentation what is the best for baby. Nursing mothers can also take the tea themselves.

Dill tea (gripe water)
- griping pains
- gas
- colic
- soothing
- menstrual problems

Fennel
Foeniculum vulgare syn. *Anethum foeniculum*

**Apiaceae
(Umbelliferae)
Carrot family**

Description: Hardy
biennial or perennial;
upright, blue–green
hollow stem, 70cm–2m
(2.5–6ft) high; finely
branched leaves;
hairless; multiple tiny
yellow flowers in large
umbels, followed by
small greenish fruit
that ripens to brown;
smells strongly of
aniseed.

Distribution: A native
of southern Europe
and SW Asia, now
cultivated widely in
hotter, drier parts of
the temperate world
as a garden and
commercial vegetable;
grows wild Down Under
(ask any New Zealand
vehicle driver).

Varieties: Florence
fennel is grown as
a vegetable for its
swollen bulb. Fennel
grown for seed is
usually called sweet
fennel, though it
reverts to the older
wilder bitter fennel. It
is available in green or
bronze forms.

Related species:
Medicinally close to
other carrot family
members, such as
anise, coriander and
dill.

Parts used: Fresh and
dried leaves, dried fruit
(seeds), root, oil from
whole plant.

Medicinally, fennel is an aromatic, warming herb, well tolerated for soothing the digestion and treating urinary and nervous disorders; it is taken for infant colic and by lactating mothers; it is a potential slimming aid, and an old remedy for inflamed eyes; as a hot or cold compress it eases headaches and migraines.

Fennel is a single species in its own genus, *foeniculum*, within the large Apiaceae family. Both the scientific and common names derive from the Latin for 'little hay', which probably refers to the feathery appearance of the dried leaves. In India its most used names translate as 'one hundred flowers' and 'the sweet one'.

Fennel's two main volatile oils influence whether it tastes more sweet or bitter. Fencone is a bitter element, which predominates in wild fennel from central Europe and Russia. Anethole is sweet-smelling, and gives the characteristic aniseed tang associated with sweet or Roman fennel, originally from the Mediterranean but now worldwide.

Sweet fennel (*Foeniculum vulgare* var. *dulce*) is the aromatic swollen-root form used in modern cooking and salads. It is sometimes earthed up, like celery, for extra blanching. The medicinal part is usually the seeds (fruits), best harvested as they start turning brown, and crushed to release the oils before being used as a tea.

Fennel is a herb of ancient repute, its uses spanning the magical and spiritual, medicinal and culinary. It was known to Old World cultures including ancient Egypt, classical Greece and Rome, India and later in China. It translocated readily to North America and Australia.

In Greek myth Prometheus is said to have stolen fire from the gods and brought it to man in the hollow stem of a mature fennel (in northern Europe wild elder was said to be the carrier plant).

Fennel was one of nine sacred herbs of the Anglo-Saxons in tenth-century manuscripts, and long after that was a protective herb in midsummer festivals. The Physicians of Myddfai, Wales wrote in the thirteenth century: 'He who sees fennel and gathers it not, is not a man but a devil.'

Use fennel for…

A key to fennel's use is the belief by Ayurvedic physicians in India that its action is to balance the body and mind, between too heating and too cooling. A modern western herbal links this

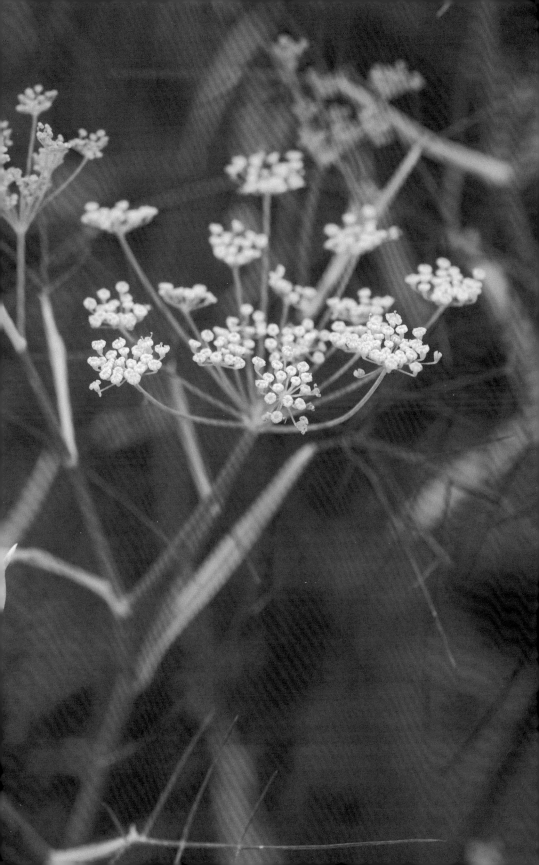

with a beautiful phrase from the medieval German abbess and herbalist, Hildegard of Bingen: 'fennel forces [a person] back into the right balance of joyfulness'.

So while fennel seeds eaten after a meal stimulate the digestion, they also stave off hunger; indeed, fennel was used on Christian fast days, as well as in old classical and some modern slimming formulas.

It was taken with stronger purging herbs to modify their harshness, and was thought to counteract

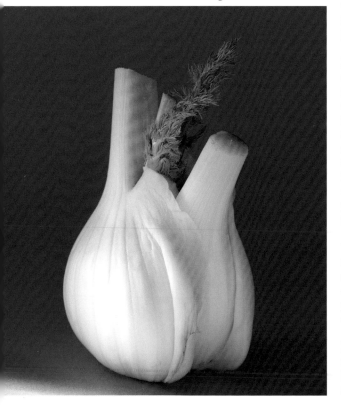

various poisons. It remains useful to sweeten rather bitter tonics in herbal formulas. In our times, the seeds boiled in milk are a good digestive and strong enough to clear coughs and bronchial stress.

Yet fennel is also gentle in tea form, and used for easing wind or colic in children (though not as mild as dill). It is a standard part of gripe water formulas, along with anise and dill. Some herbalists recommend a fennel tea bath for soothing infants, as their skin is highly permeable, while other practitioners prefer the mother to drink the fennel tea herself and pass it on in her milk.

Fennel has an old reputation as an aid in mothers' lactation, though used less nowadays than fenugreek. It also shares in fenugreek's capacity to be moistening in menopausal dryness; a fennel cream is used to stop menopausal hair growth. But, to balance the picture, large doses of fennel are best avoided in pregnancy as it is overstimulating for some mothers-to-be.

The stronger fennel root shares the diuretic and laxative qualities of parsley, meaning the root tea can be used to reduce high blood pressure and fluid retention, and ease urination and constipation.

Externally, a compress made from cold fennel tea is an ancient but still effective home remedy for treating eye inflammations (blepharitis) and conjunctivitis. It also makes a good wrinkle ointment, which is also mildly antiseptic, so protecting the skin from infection.

For an easy skin lotion, combine fennel tea with honey and yogurt, while the seeds boiled and strained make an aromatic final shampoo rinse.

Fennel bulb is essentially water, cellulose and its volatile oils, working more by aroma and taste than by actual sustenance for the plant contains few calories and vitamins, and no starches.

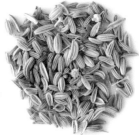

Fennel seeds should be in every family medicine chest, for they are a remedy for conditions that occur very frequently; I am speaking of griping pains and flatulence.
– Abbé Kneipp (1890s)

Abbé Kneipp's fennel in milk
The Abbé boiled 1 teaspoon **fennel seed** in a cupful of **milk** for 5–10 minutes. The result was to be drunk as hot as possible. He found it 'generally brings about a rapid improvement, [as] the warmth spreads through the body'.

Fennel ointment
Melt ½ cup **coconut oil** in a small saucepan. Grind or crush a couple of tablespoons of **fennel seed** using a spice or coffee grinder or a mortar and pestle. Add to the coconut oil and simmer gently for 15 minutes. Strain and pour into a small jar.

Fennel tea
Pour a cup of **boiling water** over 1 teaspoonful **fennel seed**. Cover and infuse for 5 minutes. Strain and drink hot. Can also be used cold as a soothing eyebath.

Seed and mint tea
Mix roughly equal parts **fennel seed**, **dill or caraway seed** and **peppermint**. Pour a cup of **boiling water** over 1 teaspoonful. Cover and infuse for 5 minutes. Strain and drink hot.

Mukhwas
Mix together 1 cup **fennel seed** and ½ cup finely **shredded coconut**, then dry-roast lightly in a pan. This mix can be ground to a powder.

This is our adaptation of a South Asian after-meal digestive aid, *mukhwas* being derived from two words meaning 'mouth' and 'smell'. Other sweet spices, sugar and peppermint oil are sometimes used in addition or instead, but the essential idea is that of an aromatic mouth- and breath-sweetener taken after food.

Abbé Kneipp's fennel in milk
- griping pains
- flatulence
- 'flu

Fennel ointment
- dry skin
- vaginal dryness
- vulval itching
- menopausal facial hair growth

Fennel tea
- colic
- griping pains
- abdominal gas
- flatulence
- indigestion
- sore eyes
- coughs

Seed & mint tea
- colic
- griping pains
- abdominal gas
- flatulence
- indigestion
- nausea
- over-eating

Mukhwas
- mouth-freshener
- digestive

Fenugreek *Trigonella foenum-graecum*

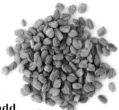

**Leguminosae
(Fabaceae)
Pea family**

Description: An
annual with trifolate
leaves, growing to
60cm (24in).
Yellow–white flowers
are followed by beaked
pods containing the
seeds.

Distribution: Grown
and widely naturalised
in Europe, the Middle
East, north Africa and
across Asia.

Parts used: Seeds,
leaves.

**From the ballad of
Lydia Pinkham**
*Mrs Jones she had no
children,/
And she loved them
very dear./
So she took three
bottles of Pinkham's,/
Now she has twins
every year.*
– An anonymous
drinking song

*… the powder of the
seede taken with a
little hony driveth
forth many noisome
humors out of the
body, mollifieth inward
Impostums and Ulcers
in the Lungs and
breasts, and
easeth the griping
paines of the intralls…*
– Parkinson (1640)

**If you have these small yellow–brown seeds
in your kitchen cupboard it is probably to add
to curries. But this ancient European and Asian herb has other roles
than as a culinary flavouring: it is effective in digestive complaints, in
balancing blood sugar in diabetes and reducing 'bad' cholesterol, as
a reproductive herb for women and for convalescence.**

The unusual name fenugreek is
an anglicised form of the Latin
for 'Greek hay', harking back to
classical Greece when the plant
was grown as a fodder crop for
animals. In modern terms it is
a nitrogen-fixing legume, and a
potential 'green manure' crop.

It is grown widely for human
consumption in the Middle East
and India. The sprouts and young
leaves are a protein-rich staple
in Yemeni cuisine, the seeds
are roasted as coffee in Egypt,
and fenugreek is an essential
ingredient of Indian curries and
curry powders. In India the seed
is known as *methi* and the dried
leaves as *kasuri methi*.

Perhaps the most surprising aspect
of fenugreek's long history (it was
used in ancient Egypt, China and
India) is its contribution to a best-
selling Victorian herbal health
formula. Lydia E. Pinkham's
Vegetable Compound dates
from mid-1870s Massachusetts,
and its original ingredients
were fenugreek (in the largest
quantity), pleurisy root, life root,

unicorn root and black cohosh.
All these are 'female herbs', and
the reason for the compound's
success was that it was the most
accessible method of self-treating
for reproductive issues. The fact
that the herbs were preserved
in 40-proof alcohol may have
contributed to its popularity.

If the name sounds familiar, it was
satirised many times, notably in
the 1968 hit by Liverpool group,
The Scaffold, as 'Lily the Pink',
with her 'medicinal compound'.

Use fenugreek for…
Fenugreek is high in accessible
mucilage (up to 30% by weight),
which soothes the whole digestive
system, from mouth to bowel.
Parkinson (1640) put it pithily:
'fenugreek cleanseth, digesteth,
dissolveth and mollifieth'.

Fenugreek's taste is pungent,
somewhat bitter, but stimulating.
In a hot infusion it will normalise
sluggish or gassy digestion, and
is calming for mouth and stomach
ulcers, and irritable bowel; it also
helps relieve constipation.

Home Remedies

An exciting area of research concerns the uses of certain herbs for reducing the 'bad' blood cholesterols LDH and VLDL; these include garlic, turmeric and fenugreek. An allied effect in fenugreek is to normalise blood sugar levels. Fenugreek is ethnobotanist James Duke's top herb for assisting in treatment of type 1 and 2 diabetes, as a home-made tea or in purchased capsules.

In Traditional Chinese Medicine fenugreek is considered a specific for treating altitude sickness.

Fenugreek is well established as a reproductive herb. Its seeds contain diosgenin, a saponin used to produce oestrogen in manufactured oral contraceptives.

Fenugreek is a remedy for reducing the discomfort of vaginal dryness at menopause, and is included in formulas for disturbed menstruation. It was once used to give breast firmness without bloating for women in harems in north Africa and the Middle East. It is used today in formulas for natural bust enlargement. Fenugreek also promotes lactation, and is a childbirth herb in India.

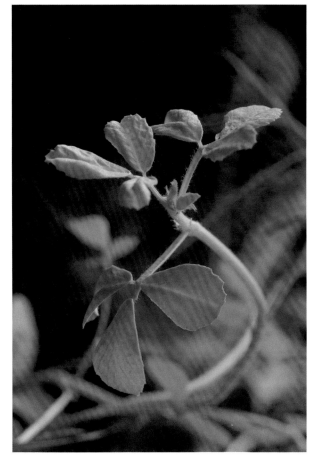

Fenugreek is nutritious as sprouts, as are fellow legumes mung beans and alfalfa, or as a soup during convalescence.

Externally, fenugreek boiled in milk makes a soothing poultice for swellings and bruises.

Caution: claims that fenugreek interferes with anti-coagulant treatments, such as warfarin, have been challenged, and it is generally regarded as a safe herb.

Fenugreek tea
- colds
- fevers
- digestive problems
- IBS
- blood sugar imbalances
- high cholesterol
- vaginal dryness
- promotes lactation
- breast enhancement
- irregular menstruation

Fenugreek tea
Use 2 teaspoons of **fenugreek seed** per cup of **boiling water**. Cover and infuse for about 3 minutes. If brewed for much longer it becomes quite bitter – perhaps more medicinal, but less pleasant to drink. Use cool as a gargle for sore throats or as a hair rinse.

Dose: drink hot and frequently to promote sweating in colds and 'flu; take 2 or 3 cups a day for chronic conditions.

Figs *Ficus carica*

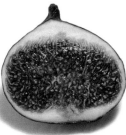

**Moraceae
Mulberry family**

Description: A deciduous tree, to 7m (21ft) tall, with smooth, pale bark, irregular forked branches, large, hand-shaped green leaves, concealed flowers and purple, white or red globular fruit.

Distribution: Native to Persia (Iran) and Asia Minor, but widespread throughout the Mediterranean; widely grown in California and other places with a Mediterranean climate.

Related species: *Ficus carica* is the one Mediterranean representative of a large genus, comprising tall forest trees, including the Asian peepul (*F. religiosa*) or Bodi tree.

Parts used: Fruit (actually a flower receptacle), latex of stems and leaves.

Taking figs for constipation is something we all know, but this ancient tree has other applications that make equally proven and effective self-medication. There is nothing to match devouring a sun-warmed, ripe fig from your own tree, and dried figs should be a staple in your kitchen cupboard.

The fig was one of the first fruits cultivated in the Near and Middle East, possibly 6000 years ago, and the fig-leaf was humanity's first 'clothing' in the creation story of Genesis. Along with olive and grape, it is the most frequently mentioned tree in the Bible.

Indeed, one of the rare herbal treatments mentioned in the Old Testament included figs. Hezekiah, king of Judah, was 'sick unto death' with a serious tumour (actually a boil), whereupon the prophet Isaiah said: 'Let them take a lump of figs, and lay it for plaister upon the boil, and he shall recover.' And he did (Isaiah 38.21).

A fig compress is still an effective treatment for skin eruptions. Similarly, when you swallow syrup of figs for constipation, you are doing something that the Egyptian pharaohs did: the Ebers manuscript, written about 1500 BC, specifies soaking fresh figs overnight in 'sweet beer' and taking the drink 'often' for this purpose.

In addition to being medicinal, figs have long been prized as an excellent and easily grown source of sugar, which when dried could be stored until the following year. Drying concentrates the nutritional value of figs, and soaking them in water or milk overnight produces an energy booster for your morning muesli, as well as preventing constipation.

In ancient Rome inferior figs were slave food and the best, for the social elite, came from Caria in present-day Turkey – the origin of the plant's scientific name. To the Spartans, figs were nourishing food for athletes, and Roman legionaries ate dried figs when marching. Pechey's herbal of 1707 states that the Roman physician Galen (AD 131–200) 'ate no other fruit, after Twenty eight Years of Age, than Figs and Raisins'.

Use figs for…
Modern usage repeats ancient wisdom, as figs remain an ingredient of jams, syrups and biscuits that are tasty and readily

absorbed. As eighteenth-century herbalist William Meyrick put it, 'This fruit is accounted grateful to the stomach, moderately nourishing, and is more easily digested than any of the other sweet fruits.' Note that too many figs can be upsetting to the stomach, as Parkinson reminded his readers in 1640 (see quote).

Apart from Adam's covering of fig-leaves, the most familiar of fig's uses has been its role as a gentle laxative for children and adults alike. It is a partner in a classic syrup made with senna (*Senna alexandrina*), a stronger purgative. Fig brings soluble fibre as well as sugar to the mixture, is demulcent – soothes the intestines – and makes an unpleasant but effective remedy more palatable.

Externally, fresh or slightly roasted figs give relief when placed, as hot as can be borne, on gum or tooth abscesses, and a fig mouthwash or gargle can be made by boiling half a dozen fruits in a litre of water or milk until soft. The same fluid soothes a cough or bronchitis.

Mashed figs applied to hot eruptions of the skin, like boils, or to burns, in a compress can be as effective today as for King Hezekiah. A Coptic remedy of some 3000 years ago adds fig leaves to natron (hydrated sodium carbonate), sulphur and honey to make a rub for inflamed skin.

The white latex of fig branches and leaves can be applied on warts, bites and stings, but it is toxic and must not be used internally; it can also cause an allergic reaction to the sun. Pechey cautioned in 1707: 'The Juice of the Fig-tree is very biting, and may be reckoned among the Causticks; and may be used to cure Warts, and other sordid Excrescencies of the Skin.'

Figs are restorative, and the best food that can be taken by those who are brought low by long sickness. … professed wrestlers and champions in times past fed with figs.
– Pliny (1st century AD)

… if they be eaten while they are fresh and greene, they loosen the belly, but doe somewhat trouble the stomacke: the dryed Figges doe heate the stomacke, and cause thirst, yet they nourish and are good for the throate, and arteries, the reignes [kidneys] and bladder…
– Parkinson (1640)

A friendly syrup of figs
Take some 50g (about 2oz) each of **dried figs**, **raisins** and **barley** grain. Boil in about a litre of water (1.75 pt) for 15 minutes; then add a small handful of **licorice powder** to taste. Keep cooking for 15 minutes more. Allow to cool down and strain, retaining the liquid.
Take a small cup morning and evening as a laxative. This recipe was 'prescribed by doctors as a capital demulcent', noted Fernie in 1895.

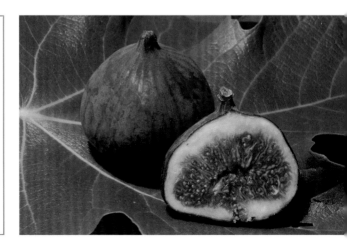

Garlic *Allium sativum*

Liliaceae
Lily family

Description: A bulbous perennial onion usually grown as an annual, producing numerous 'cloves' or bulblets.

Distribution: Garlic is native to central Asia but now grown worldwide; it needs cold weather to produce bulblets.

Related species: There are over 700 species in the onion genus, many of them used for food and medicine. These include onion (*A. cepa*), chives (*A. schoenoprasum*), Asian onion (*A. fistulosum*) and leek (*A. porrum*).

Parts used: Bulblets and green tops.

No other herb comes close to the multiple system actions of garlic, its antibiotic activity, and immune-potentiating power.
– Buhner (1999)

Now, bolt down these cloves of garlic. … Well primed with garlic, you will have greater mettle for the fight!
– Aristophanes (fourth century BC)

Garlic is known for its antibiotic properties. It is also a circulatory tonic, increasing blood flow and reducing blood pressure and lowering levels of harmful cholesterol, thereby protecting against heart attack and stroke. Garlic improves digestion, stimulating secretion of digestive enzymes and bile, and helps maintains a healthy gut flora. It also clears catarrh and has an affinity for the respiratory tract.

Garlic has been a food and medicine for thousands of years. Many prescriptions of the ancient Egyptians included garlic for treatment of ailments from infections to physical weakness. Khnoum Khoufouf, builder of one of the oldest pyramids, in 4500 BC gave all his labourers a clove of garlic each morning to keep up their strength and health.

The ancient Greeks used it freely, and athletes at the Olympic Games ate garlic to enhance their performance. The Romans gave it to both soldiers and workmen. Garlic was by no means limited to Europe, however. Ayurvedic physicians in India prescribed it for rheumatism and to prevent heart disease, and in Japan and China from ancient times it was a remedy for high blood pressure.

The English 'garlic' is reputedly from the Anglo-Saxon for 'spear plant', perhaps referring to the shape of its leaves or garlic being soldier fare. Culpeper said garlic was ruled by Mars, god of war.

We all know that garlic protects us against vampires. In many cultures, from old Asia to old Europe, garlic has been used to ward off the evil eye, witches, sorcerers, spells and evil spirits. Physically, it still strengthens our defences against a wide range of 'evil' influences, from infections and poisons to high blood pressure and the risk of stroke and heart attack.

Like other powerful herbs, garlic has a mixed reputation. Its sulphurous smell had associations with the devil. In England and other places where garlic has not been much a part of traditional cooking, the odour on the breath is considered offensive. Neither of us had fresh garlic until we were in our twenties – garlic salt was then the only form you could buy.

In India, yogis, orthodox Hindus and Jains reject onions or garlic in their food as too stimulating, saying they root the consciousness more firmly in the body and interfere with meditation.

On the other hand, garlic is much enjoyed elsewhere in sauces such as skorthalia in Greece, guacamole in Mexico, humous in the Middle East, pesto in Italy and aïoli in Spain and France. We grow some as perennial clumps and harvest the green tops every spring. They are among our earliest spring greens, and provide a milder garlic flavour than the bulbs.

Use garlic for...

Garlic was used in both the First and Second World Wars to treat battle wounds, preventing sepsis and gangrene. Garlic is effective against both gram-positive and gram-negative bacteria, while having the enviable quality of being harmless to our normal, beneficial gut bacteria. This is unlike modern broad-spectrum antibiotics, which wipe everything out. Garlic is known to be effective against fungal, parasitic and viral infections.

For its antibiotic properties, garlic needs to be used raw. It is only once it is crushed that the powerful antibiotic allicin is formed, and the sulphury smell released. One of the most palatable

Garlic then have power to save from death,/ Bear with it though it maketh unsavoury breath,/ And scorn not garlic like some that think / It only maketh men wink and drink and stink.
– after Harington (1607)

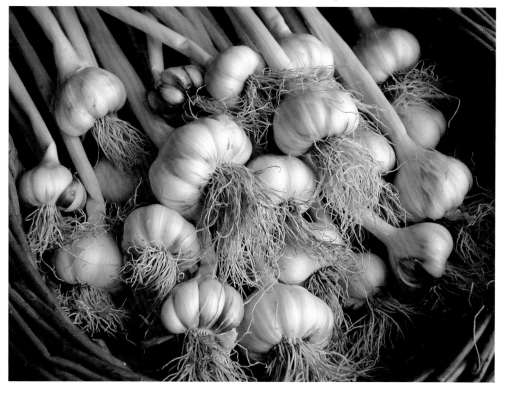

Freshly harvested garlic

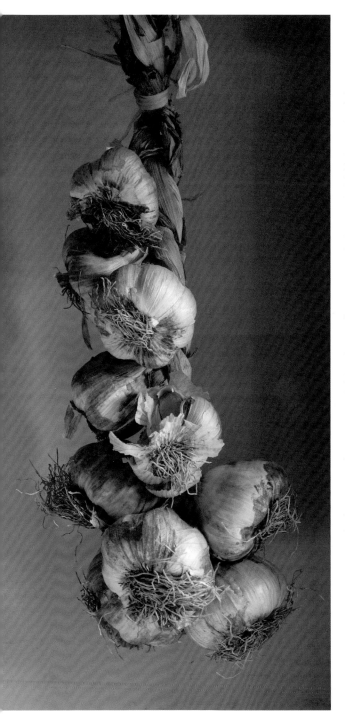

ways to take it raw is in garlic butter or blended with oil in a salad dressing. Sauces with raw garlic are tasty medicine. Julie's father never liked garlic until she made him fresh basil and garlic pesto, which was so tasty that he forgot about the antisocial aroma.

People who worry about this can take odourless garlic capsules, which still have a protective value for the heart and circulation, but are not as strong in antibiotic effect. Chewing on fresh parsley or a cardamom pod readily clears the breath after eating garlic.

Applied to the soles of the feet it is an old remedy for chest infections. Mix it with some oil or fat first so that it will not burn the skin, then apply and wrap the feet warmly for half an hour before rinsing off.

Garlic has been found to reduce blood sugar levels in diabetics. It also lowers cholesterol levels, reduces high blood pressure and thins the blood. In fact, people on blood-thinning medication need to be careful when adding garlic to the diet. Garlic exerts a powerful protective action on the circulation and the heart, and also reduces the risk of stroke.

Remember that garlic, especially raw, is a hot herb so it may be too heating for some people. If this is so, try substituting milder leeks, which are less heating but still have many of the beneficial qualities of garlic.

Garlic comes ready-protected with a double white skin-membrane, one for each clove and one for the whole head. These keep the smells in until the cloves are cut or crushed. Note that old cloves may get a black fungus or go hard and empty, so choose fresh, plump cloves to buy and keep. Best of all, grow your own!

The common names 'clown's treacle' and 'poor man's treacle' are references to garlic's home-cure status, a 'treacle' being an anti-dote to poisons, stings and bites.
– Hemphill (2006)

... we absolutely forbid it entrance into our Salleting [salad making], by reason of its intolerable Rankness. ... To be sure,'tis not for Ladies Palats, nor those who court them, farther than to permit a light touch on the Dish, with a Clove thereof.
– Evelyn (1699)

Garlic honey

Peel a **whole head of garlic**. Mince finely by chopping or squeezing through a garlic press. Put in a mortar and pound until the garlic begins to go transparent. Spoon into a jar with 225g (½lb) of **honey**. Stir well, seal and label.

Dose: half a teaspoonful daily as a tonic or preventative. For acute infections, take half a teaspoonful up to six times daily. This can be taken directly, or taken with ginger and lemon tea or cider vinegar. For infants and young children, rub onto the soles of the feet.

Garlic honey can also be used directly on the skin for bites, and as a wound dressing for cuts and grazes.

Four thieves' vinegar

There are as many recipes for thieves' vinegar as there are versions of the myth. Basically, in early eighteenth-century France four thieves were arrested for stealing from the homes of dead plague victims. They were given their lives and freedom in exchange for the recipe they used to keep free of the disease. The recipe was added to the official French pharmacopoeia, and it is still sold today as *Le vinaigre des quatre voleurs*.

The essential ingredients are **vinegar** and **garlic**, and then you can add other aromatic herbs and spices as available: **rosemary**, **sage**, **oregano**, **mint**, **lavender**, **cinnamon**, **cloves** etc. Some people like to throw in an **onion**, and **horseradish** or **hot chillies**.

It is worth making quite a big batch. Use roughly equal parts of crushed garlic and each of a selection of four or five other aromatic herbs. Put in a jar large enough to hold them and cover with red wine vinegar (or cider vinegar). Seal and put in a warm place for two or three weeks, then strain and bottle for use.

Your thieves' vinegar can be used several ways:
• take a teaspoonful several times a day
• add to salad dressings
• use a tablespoon in the bath
• use topically as an antiseptic on the skin
• use as a topical spray for disinfecting kitchen surfaces.

Garlic honey
• colds
• fevers
• coughs
• infections
• cuts and grazes

Four thieves' vinegar
• antiseptic
• prevents infection
• aids digestion
• colds
• 'flu
• gastric infections

Ginger Zingiber officinale

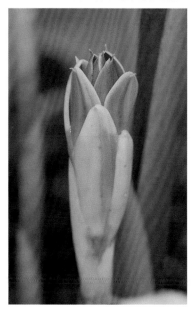

Ginger is the best natural remedy for nausea of all types. It is also excellent for strengthening weak digestion, improving poor circulation and warming any cold conditions of the body. It clears phlegm from the lungs and induces sweating, making it a beneficial treatment for colds and other infections.

Zingiberaceae
Ginger family

Description: A deciduous tropical perennial, with a thick, finger-like aromatic root or rhizome.

Distribution: Native to tropical Asia, and widely grown in the tropics worldwide.

Related species: There are around 100 species in the ginger family, and many of them are used in cooking and medicine, including cardamom, galangal and turmeric.

Parts used: Rhizome.

Nose, nose, jolly red nose, who gave thee this jolly red nose?/ Nutmegs and ginger, cinnamon and cloves,/ And they gave me this jolly red nose.
– Beaumont & Fletcher (1609), based on an older drinking song

As everyone knows, ginger is 'hot'! A 'ginger group' is one that gets things moving. Technically, the rhizome of this tropical plant is pungent and sweet, but it is ginger's warming effects on the body, in food and medicine (and aphrodisiac use) that has made it one of the chief spices of trade from the East since ancient times.

The English name is derived from the Sankrit term *Singabera*, which became Latin *Zingiber* and later 'ginger'.

In tropical countries, fresh ginger is predominantly used in cooking while temperate pantries are more likely to have powdered dry ginger or crystallised ginger on hand. In the last two decades, though, fresh ginger has become more widely available worldwide, with China, Thailand and Brazil the main exporters of the beige-coloured roots found in our shops.

In Ayurveda, India's ancient system of healing, ginger is effectively a universal medicine, benefiting all people and all diseases. It increases digestive fire, clears toxins from the body and improves circulation – three key actions that help most conditions.

Ginger has been cultivated for so long that it rarely grows as a wild plant. It was a prized import to the Roman empire, where it was primarily used as a medicine.

In England in the late Middle Ages ginger was almost as common as pepper. By this time, preserved ginger as well as the dried herb were being imported, and it was widely used to make gingerbread.

Recipes for gingerbread were tremendously varied, from medieval recipes with honey and breadcrumbs to later ginger cakes and biscuits. Gingerbread was often elaborately decorated or shaped by intricately carved wooden moulds. Gold leaf was sometimes used to decorate gingerbread – hence the saying 'gilt on the gingerbread'.

Use ginger for…

Ginger is the best remedy for nausea of all types, including morning sickness in pregnancy, travel sickness and nausea caused by chemotherapy treatment. You may find nibbling a ginger cookie or sipping a ginger beer is enough to alleviate feelings of sickness, or try chewing crystallised ginger.

For a stronger dose, stir a teaspoonful of ginger powder into a mug of hot water and sip that, or make the ginger decoction given overleaf. Alternatively, use the powder in empty capsules, bought from health shops or herbalists.

This is the herbalist's best friend.
– Pole (2006)

Ginger is such a powerful stimulant that when used in excess, it can detoxify your system bringing out too much junk too fast.
– Dewey (1996)

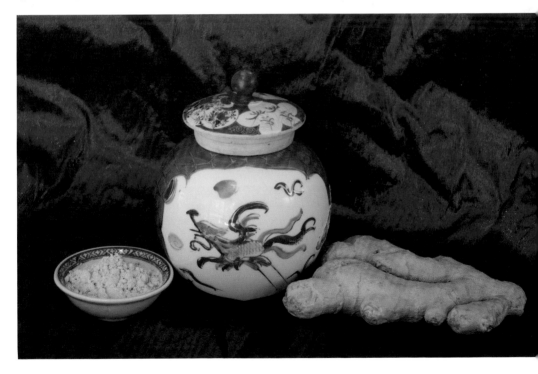

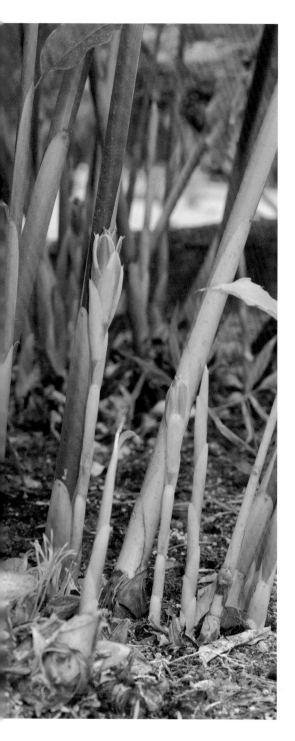

Studies show that ginger is effective against the bacteria that cause diarrhoea and digestive upsets.

Ginger is an excellent remedy for colds and fevers, as it promotes sweating and helps clear mucus from the throat and lungs. Drink ginger tea and have a hot ginger bath at the first sign of a cold.

As we age, our digestive processes tend to slow down, often resulting in queasiness, nausea, gas and bloating. Ginger is superb at stimulating digestive secretions, improving transit time of food through the alimentary canal and relieving these symptoms. It also stimulates circulation and helps keep the blood thin, protecting the heart and warming cold hands and feet, something else we need to deal with as we age. It can also help maintain mental alertness.

Ginger is effective in several ways for arthritis. By improving digestion, it helps eliminate the toxins that can build up from improperly digested food and affect the joints. Used externally and internally, it stimulates circulation, warming stiff and painful joints and helping eliminate waste products. Ginger also helps to reduce inflammation.

Fresh ginger and dried ginger can be used interchangeably for many conditions, but be aware that dried ginger is much hotter than the fresh rhizome. When ginger is dried the gingerols it contains transform to shogoals, which are more heating and have more of a blood-thinning effect.

Incorporating ginger into your daily diet will help maintain health and protect you against chronic degenerative illnesses.

Ginger tea

Grate about an inch (2.5cm) of **fresh ginger root** into a small saucepan with a couple of cups of **water** in it. Bring to a boil, then turn down the heat and simmer gently for about ten minutes. Strain and drink.

Ginger and onion soup

Chop up three **onions**. Sauté in a little oil until transparent, then add 3 cups of **water** or vegetable stock.

Add 3 teaspoonfuls **grated fresh ginger.** Then, add 2 cloves **garlic,** pressed or chopped finely**,** 1 fresh **chilli**, chopped finely, or 1 teaspoonful dried **chilli powder** and 1 small stick **cinnamon** or 1 teaspoonful **cinnamon powder**.

Bring to the boil and simmer gently for a few minutes, then serve.

Hot healing oil

Warm ½ cup **olive oil** with a 1-inch (2.5cm) piece fresh **ginger,** chopped finely (or 2 teaspoonfuls **ginger powder),** 1 or 2 **chillies**, chopped finely (or 1 teaspoonful **chilli powder**) in a small saucepan for half an hour.

You can also add in **minced garlic, mustard powder, black pepper** or **horseradish**, depending on what heating herbs you have available.

The warmed oil can be used straightaway if needed, otherwise pour the whole mixture into a jar and let it brew for a week or two before straining and bottling. Rub into sore or stiff muscles and joints several times a day as needed.

Ginger bath

Adding dry ginger to a hot bath stimulates sweating and the elimination of toxins. It's great at the first signs of a cold or fever, though be careful not to exceed the dose or you may detoxify too quickly for comfort.

Put 4 tablespoons of **ginger powder** in a sock or tie it in a piece of cloth, then place it under the running hot water. When you get in the bath, squeeze it to extract more of the ginger. To amplify the effect, drink a cup of ginger tea while you are in the bath. Stay in the hot bath for about 20 minutes, then get out and go to bed.

Ginger poultice

Mix equal parts **ginger powder** and **cornmeal or flour,** and add enough **water** to make a thick paste. Apply over a boil, cover with a piece of plastic and bandage in place. Applying heat over the poultice with a hot water bottle or heating pad will bring the boil to maturation even faster.

Ginger tea
- nausea
- weak digestion
- menstrual cramps
- morning sickness
- travel sickness
- poor circulation
- colds & coughs

Ginger & onion soup
- colds
- chills
- 'flu & fevers
- respiratory infections
- circulation

Hot healing oil
- muscle aches
- stiffness
- arthritic pain
- ganglions
- backache
- sports injuries

Ginger bath
- colds
- fevers
- chills
- detoxing

Ginger poultice
- boils

Cautions: Ginger is very safe as a medicine, but if you are a 'hot' person, dried ginger may be too heating and stimulating – use the fresh rhizome instead. If you are on blood-thinning medication such as warfarin, add ginger gradually to your diet. Note that high doses of dried ginger may reduce the dose needed of your medication.

Honey *Mel*

Honey as food, honey as medicine: it is superb both ways, a wonderful standby in kitchen medicine. Antiseptic, soothing and nutritious, it brings us the benefits of nature's premier herbalist, the bee. Age-old in wound applications, it has come under new scrutiny as a possible weapon against hospital 'superbugs', including MRSA.

Honey is produced by the honey bee from nectar from plants, and stored in a hive made of wax. The European honey bee is *Apis mellifera*. There are about 20,000 known species of bees but only seven species of honey bee, all in the genus Apis. Some other bees also make and store honey.

A teaspoonful of honey is said to be a honey bee's lifework.

A hive of useful products
In addition to honey, honey bees produce:
Royal jelly: food for all infant bees and for queens through their lives: nutritious, rejuvenates the human hormonal system, improves disease resistance, adds weight.
Propolis: resins used to protect the hive from infection and a powerful antibiotic.
Pollen: nutrient-rich, promotes well-being and resistance to infection.
Wax: beeswax candles are still the ecclesiastical choice.

Caution: It is generally recommended that infants under a year of age not be given honey because of a risk of botulism.

In an old Muslim story a princess was ill. A wise man said she would recover only if she were given a thousand plants. This caused consternation until a herb seller heard about the problem. 'Give her honey,' she advised, 'for this comes from a thousand plants.' The princess soon recovered.

Honey may be a rich blend of the nectar of many plants or few, or a single species, like Scottish heather or New Zealand manuka honey. In each case the complex biochemistry of a plant's nectar is transformed in the stomachs of worker bees into sugars of honey, glucose and fructose.

This is wonderful alchemy, and man has always taken advantage of honey – as in a 10,000-year-old rock painting of two women (depicted in the nude, carrying a ladder) collecting honey from wild bees in Valencia, Spain or Sumerian clay tablets 4000 years old inscribing the first honey laws.

Bees provided man's earliest light, the beeswax used in candles, and

his main source of sweetness, their honey. One of the first alcohols was mead, a drink of fermented honey, the name originating in a Sanskrit term, *madhu*. A land flowing with milk and honey, in the Old Testament phrase, was rich indeed, with a diet that could sustain people for months.

Honey has been used medicinally in most cultures through recorded history, although in the West in the mid-twentieth century it was discarded in favour of antibiotics. In more recent years, however, the notion of unpasteurised and unheated medicinal honeys has gained a following. One of the drivers in this rediscovery is the success of honey in combating drug-resistant wound infections.

The so-called 'superbugs', group *A. streptococcus* and methicillin-resistant *Staphylococcus aureus* (MRSA), are the scourge of modern hospitals, and the use of honey in treating them is being actively researched, in Germany, Australia, New Zealand and the UK.

Use honey for…

The 'father of western medicine', Hippocrates (460–377 BC), saw honey as both medicine and food, and used honey mixed with water – in his words, a hydromel – for nearly all ailments he encountered. It is reputed that at Hippocrates' death wild bees swarmed on his tomb and took up residence there. Honey from this nest was said to have amazing healing properties.

Honey is predigested in the bee, and humans – particularly those who are sick – can absorb it unusually quickly, in half an hour. Fructose and glucose, the forms of sugar that predominate in honey, at some 30 to 40% each, taste as sweet as sucrose, with the same calories. This means that honey is not a slimming alternative to sugar, and too much can damage your teeth as well as overcome you with sweetness.

Shakespeare put it well: '… They surfeited with honey and began / To loathe the taste of sweetness, whereof a little / More than a little is by much too much.' Honey should not be taken by the obese and people with diabetes.

Note too that more than moderate heating will denature honey's chemistry, so heated blended honey is not as medicinal as unheated forms. So, when using it in teas and cooking, avoid boiling it. On the other hand, caramelised honey makes a delicious glaze on figs, ham etc.

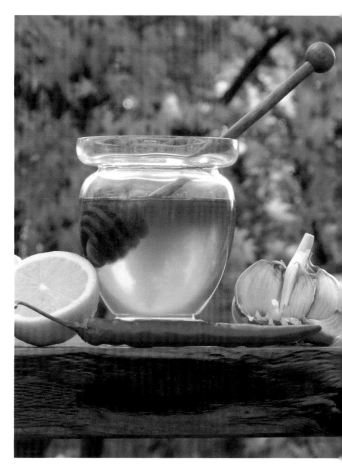

Honey is highly antiseptic and antitoxic, making it a 'times immemorial' wound and skin healer. It is hygroscopic, ie absorbs moisture, and denies pathogens at the source of an infection the liquid environment they need to thrive. Honey is said to be 'drawing', in cases of poisons or infected wounds. It was put to this life-saving use in the trenches of the First World War.

… the honeybee, Apis mellifera, *our planet's premier herbalists and medicine-makers.*
– Green (2000)

Instead of dirt and poison [said the bees] *we have rather chosen to fill our hives with honey and wax; thus furnishing mankind with the two noblest of things, which are sweetness and light.*
– Swift (1704)

To make mead
An eighteenth-century Norfolk recipe (verbatim)
To a pound of Honey 5 pints Water and a ¼ pound of Raisons stoned let 'em all boyl together an hour & scum it well put in a Tub and when cold put in a Toast spread with yest on both sides and cover it close till the next Day then lade it up and down & let it stand two Days and then Tun it up.

More honey herbalism
An **oxymel** is a herbal honey with vinegar, and is used where an intense herb needs a carrier for absorption, eg garlic or cayenne. Apple cider vinegar sweetened with honey is a home remedy for 'flu and arthritis.

An **electuary** (or conserve) is a delivery mechanism for difficult-to-swallow dried herbs, eg black pepper for hayfever. The powdered herb is mixed with a spoonful of honey, rolled into a ball and swallowed.

Honey is moist, lubricating and soothing for inflammation, especially of the digestive and respiratory tracts. The classic western use of honey is for relieving dryness and soreness in the throat, and for coughs and problems with swallowing. It is the professional singer's standby for hoarseness. The honey is either eaten, diluted in warm water, taken with lemon or made into herb honey, such as sage.

Honey is nutritious and gives energy while allaying nervous tension, hence is excellent for those who are overworked, depressed or convalescing. It can be taken before sleep as a mild sedative. Be aware that it is also slightly laxative in some people, supporting the liver and kidneys if out of balance.

At home a suggested remedy for acne is to cover the pimple with honey and a sticky plaster overnight – the honey keeps it sterile while raising the sore pimple; bee stings can be disinfected with honey; fresh bruises can be rubbed with honey, while for burns honey is a speed healer, producing an airless, dry, protected environment where the micro-organisms cannot reproduce. In such external treatments thicken too-runny honey with cornflour (cornstarch).

Herbal honeys

Honey is better for us than sucrose taken as refined sugar because honey contains non-sugar elements from the original plant sources and does not upset the body's mineral balance as pure sugar can. Herbalists amplify this in herbal honeys or syrups, oxymels and electuaries.

The **herb** of choice, such as sage or thyme, is warmed at low temperature with **honey** in a saucepan for up to an hour, and then strained and bottled. The properties of the herb combine with those of honey, making herbal honeys particularly good for throat problems.

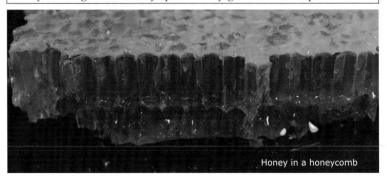
Honey in a honeycomb

Lemon *Citrus limon, C. medica* var. *limonum*

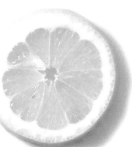

Lemon is a remarkably versatile fruit, offering sour, slightly sweet, bitter, acid and astringent tastes; each of these qualities widens its medicinal and culinary value. Known universally for its vitamin C content and action on scurvy and as a domestic cold and 'flu treatment, it has other applications as varied as arteriosclerosis and anorexia, and supports the immune system and liver.

The name 'lemon' comes from north Indian *limu* or *ninbu*, via Arabic *limun* and Latin *limon*, the small changes encapsulating many centuries in the plant's botanical journey from Indian origin, Arab cultivation and trade to wider scientific acceptance.

Lemons became widely cultivated in southern Europe and north Africa in areas controlled by the Arabs, but the fruit remained rare and expensive in northern parts of the continent beyond medieval times. Louis XIV's court in France later popularised the use of lemon in cooked sauces and refreshing drinks, and its many culinary and medicinal possibilities belatedly began to be recognised.

Early in its history, lemon was used more often as a preservative and to render questionable meat safe to eat. Medicinally it developed a reputation for dealing with poisons and intestinal worms. Today's squeeze of lemon on freshly opened oysters or shellfish echoes such older preventative uses.

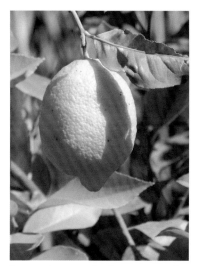

Lemon's strength of action is still valued in commercial cleaning agents as an antibacterial and germicidal; it is known to kill many dangerous bacilli, including those for typhoid and cholera, and is a general kitchen antiseptic. In older herbals lemon was recommended for treating stone in the kidney and bladder and for gravel in the liver; these uses, interestingly, still persist in Ayurveda but less so in western herbal tradition.

Rutaceae
Rue family

Description: A small tree, 3–6m (10–20ft) high, with irregular branches and thorns, evergreen pale green and oval leaves, clustered white and pink flowers, and the familiar ovoid fruit, about 8cm (3in) long, pale yellow, skin pitted with oil glands and an acidic pale yellow pulp.

Habitat: Subtropical, semi-desert areas; largely cultivated.

Distribution: Native to N India, Burma and SW China and still wild there; widely cultivated in the Mediterranean, California and places with similar climate.

Related species: Citron (*C. medica*), lime (*C. aurantiifolia*), bergamot orange (*C. aurantium* var. *bergamia*).

Parts used: Fruit, peel (commercially *Limonis cortex*), juice (*L. succus*), oil (*Oleum limonis*).

My living [diocese] *in Yorkshire was so far out of the way, that it was actually twelve miles from a lemon.*
– Rev. Sydney Smith (early nineteenth century)

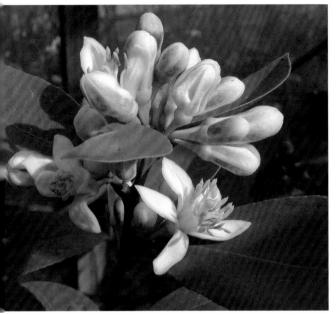

The exquisite flowers of the lemon tree, like a magnolia with attitude

It is probable that the lemon is the most valuable of all fruit for preserving health.
– Mrs Grieve (1931)

The presence of lemons in the kitchen should not deter us from viewing this fruit as a fully-fledged botanical remedy.
– Holmes (1989)

at sea – an amount that modern research finds supplies a good proportion of the recommended daily allowance of vitamin C for a healthy adult.

Use lemons for...

Lemons are often identified in a negative way with sourness: in modern terms a bad deal is a 'lemon' and a 'sour look' isn't a happy one. But this maligns a remarkably versatile fruit: lemon is also bitter, acid and slightly sweet; each of these qualities widens its medicinal and culinary significance.

Starting from the outside, the peel or rind is pitted with glands, containing mainly the essential oil limonene. This is bitter, antiseptic and antibacterial. Dried lemon rind is sold as 'lemon zest', and it retains the oils. Take note that most lemons sold are waxed: if you plan to use the peel medicinally, try to source organic and unwaxed fruit.

And what of lemon and scurvy? In this potentially fatal condition the body's collagen collapses, connective tissues and blood vessel walls leak, and widespread internal bleeding follows, most evident in swollen gums and teeth falling out, and the liver and immune system fail. The main sufferers were sailors and soldiers deprived of fresh fruit and vegetables, and citrus was long considered an effective preventative and cure, centuries before vitamins were identified.

After endless campaigning, in 1795 the Admiralty made it mandatory for all British sailors to be issued with an ounce of lemon juice each per day after ten days

The white pith is also bitter, but the fleshy pulp contains some 5–6% citric acid and also 3% sugar. This sweet undertone explains why lemon juice can heighten the taste of other fruit, vegetables and fish. The flesh contains most of lemon's vitamin C, and its supply of vitamin A, but it is the pith that most strengthens the blood vessels.

Everybody is aware that lemon is a remedy to take when a cold looms, its high vitamin C improving resistance to respiratory infection, as well as cutting mucus. Lemon is equally protective for stomach infections, poor circulation and, especially, arteriosclerosis. Gargling diluted lemon juice is a zingy way to treat a sore throat.

What makes lemon particularly valuable is that, despite being a source of citric acid and the acidic vitamin C, once lemon juice is digested its action is alkalising for the body. This is why it is used for treating rheumatic conditions that are typified by overacidity.

Lemon strongly reinforces the body in those areas that scurvy weakens. So it strengthens the gums, is healing for mouth ulcers and is a remedy for whitening the teeth; it reinforces connective tissue and blood vessel walls; it supports the immune system and the liver. Its sourness helps stimulate bile and enhances appetite. This last quality makes lemon good for treating anorexia, nausea and morning and travel sickness.

Add in that it makes a delicious, thirst-quenching drink (the first lemonade recipe is said to date from eleventh-century Egypt), enhances any cooked food and is tonic and nourishing, and lemon's versatility becomes clear.

Lemon juice is refrigerant and antiscorbutic, and is exceedingly useful in forming agreeable and refreshing beverages, for allaying thirst, and in febrile and inflammatory complaints. These drinks may be given in the form of lemonade, or lemon juice may be added to barley water. ... Lemon juice is one of the best remedies we possess in scurvy, acting both as a prophylactic and curative agent.
– Bentley & Trimen (1880)

Lemon and sage drink
Steep in 2 cups boiling water for 15 minutes: 2 teaspoons grated **organic lemon rind**, 1 teaspoon **sage leaf**, 1 teaspoon **thyme leaf**. Strain and add the **juice of half a lemon**, and **honey** to taste.

Take two or three times a day, hot or cold as you prefer.

Lemon and ginger tea
Put 4 or 5 slices of **fresh ginger** in a teapot or mug, add **boiling water** and then squeeze in the juice from a **wedge of lemon** and add a spoonful of **honey**.

This tea is refreshing, zingy, warming and fights off colds. It is a great drink first thing every morning, and can be drunk anytime just because it tastes good!

Nimbu lemonade
Stir ½ teaspoonful **sugar** and ¼ teaspoonful **rock salt** into a glass of **water** until dissolved. Add the **juice of half a lemon**, and **crushed ice** as desired. Mint leaves can also be added.

Refreshing and thirst-quenching on a hot day, this drink is a tasty oral rehydration solution to replenish electrolytes lost by sweating.

Lemon & sage drink
• coughs
• colds
• sore throat
• bronchitis

Lemon & ginger tea
• coughs
• colds
• sore throat
• sluggish digestion

Nimbu lemonade
• hot weather
• dehydration

Mushrooms _Agaricus bisporus, Lentinus edodes,_ etc

Mushrooms have come out of the shadows! The immune-support and anti-cancer capacities of medicinal mushrooms, specifically shiitake and reishi, are recognised but new research suggests that the ordinary white button mushroom has similar potential.

Description:
Mushroom is not an exact classification, but essentially is a macrofungus with an above-ground fruiting body. At least 14,000 mushroom species have been named to date, but it is estimated there may be 140,000 in total, of which many could be of future benefit to humanity.

Leading medicinal mushrooms: Maitake (_Grifola frondosa_), reishi (_Ganoderma lucidum_), shiitake (_Lentinus edodes_).

Many phantasticall people doe greatly delight to eat of the earthly excrescences called Mushrums. They are convenient for no season, age or temperament.
– Venner (1620)

… the best advice [from a mushroom hunter of fifty years] _of all is: if in doubt do not collect a mushroom and never, ever, eat anything you cannot identify with certainty._
– Jordan & Wheeler (1995)

The names of fungi are the first delight: an ABC of eatable wild British varieties includes amethyst deceiver, blewit and boletus, cep and chanterelle. The most popular commercial eating mushrooms also trip off the tongue: chestnut, crimini, enoki, porcini, portobello. Let us add another name: the origin of 'toadstool' is arguably German _Todesstuhl_, death's chair.

It gives you pause, but just as not all wild mushrooms are edible, not all toadstools are poisonous. Safe mushroom-foraging depends on accurate identification, and there are dangers in getting it wrong.

When I first became a vegetarian [Matthew recalls], I was amazed and delighted that something so vibrant and alive as a mushroom was in my diet. They have never done me any harm that I can recall, but until working with Julie on this book I hadn't realised they were actually doing me a lot of good, over and above the taste.

We are talking ordinary white button or stalked mushrooms here (_Agaricus bisporus_, technically), and also the delicious but medicinal

shiitake (_Lentinus edodes_), which these days can be bought in supermarkets. Not the medicinal reishi (_Ganoderma lucidum; ling zhi_ in China), however: Julie says ruefully, 'I have ruined a mushroom soup by adding even a little reishi – it was so bitter.'

Use mushrooms for…
Research in Japan and China has established over the last half century that shiitake and reishi are strongly immune-supporting and display anti-cancer activity.

Shiitake has natural interferon, which induces an immune response against cancer and viral diseases, notably gastric and cervical or colorectal cancer. It also decreases fat and blood cholesterol, and modifies side effects of chemotherapy.

Reishi contains adenosine, which inhibits platelet formation and helps reduce high blood pressure. It works powerfully in treating HIV / AIDS, ME and side effects of chemotherapy.

What is fascinating is that new research suggests shop-bought

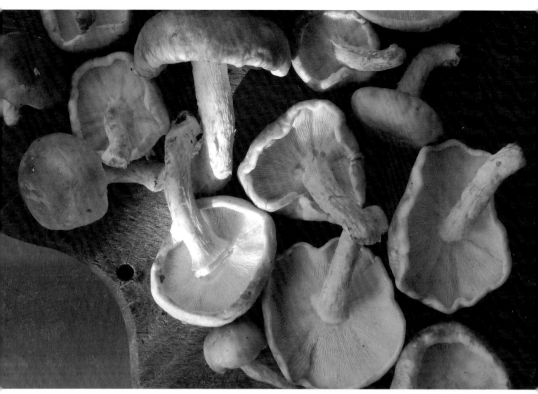

Shiitake mushrooms

mushrooms share, to a greater extent that hitherto realised, the immune-supporting and cancer-treating qualities of the explicitly medicinal mushrooms. For example, a 2009 study of 2000 Chinese women found that those who ate fresh mushrooms daily were 64% less likely to develop breast cancer; those who combined daily mushrooms with green tea reduced their risk by 90%. A 2008 paper reported in vitro trials of white button mushrooms enhancing maturation of bone marrow antigen cells. Other research is ongoing into mushroom's antibacterial, liver-protective, hypoglycaemic and immunomodulating potential.

[Shiitake contains lentinan] ... *the most powerful natural immune stimulant and restorative known.* – Bartram (1995)

Shiitake is the most delicious medicine on the planet, and you should grow your own. – Hobbs (2009)

Immune-boosting soup

Take a dozen or so **shiitake mushrooms**: use fresh if you can buy them or soak dried ones in water until soft. Slice and set aside. Chop 1 small **onion**, slice 1 **carrot** and slice 1 **potato**. Heat olive oil in a pan, sauté the mushrooms, then add the onion. As onions brown add in carrot and potato, plus 1 clove chopped **garlic** and a thumbnail of grated **ginger**. Add more oil as needed to brown all the vegetables, then add **stock** or **water** (quantity depending on whether a more solid or liquid result is desired). Bring to boil, add **soy sauce** or **miso** to taste, and / or **salt** and **pepper**. Simmer for 10 minutes and serve hot.

Caution
Eating shop-bought mushrooms is safe, but in case of mushroom poisoning from wild sources, the home remedies most readily to hand include swallowing fresh lemon juice, mustard powder, grated nutmeg or salt water in order to induce vomiting.

Mustard
Brassica alba, B. hirta, Sinapis alba **White mustard**; *B. nigra, S. nigra* **Black mustard**; *B. juncea* **Brown, Indian or Chinese mustard**

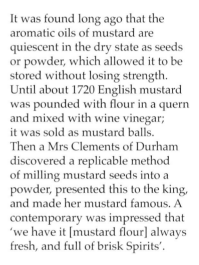

Brassicaceae
Cabbage family

Description: White mustard is an annual of about 1m (3ft) tall, while black mustard can grow up to three times higher; both have yellow flowers, but in white varieties the seed pods are longer, have a seeded 'beak' and larger rounded seeds; black types have shortish pods, with seedless 'beak' and twice as many smallish black seeds.

Distribution: White and black mustards are cultivated in temperate Europe and North America, and also grow wild; brown mustard is native to India and China and is cultivated there and other temperate areas.

Related species: Many wild Brassicas are mustards or have similar pungency, including charlock (*Sinapis arvensis*), hedge mustard (*Sisymbrium officinale*); also garden cress (*Lepidium sativum*), garden rocket (*Eruca sativa*).

Parts used: Seeds, green foliage, volatile oil.

Mustard's biting and heating nature is used to advantage to flavour and aid digestion of cooked food. The same qualities make it a convenient and effective bath and chest poultice to relieve 'cold' conditions.

Both black and white mustard were known in ancient Egypt and in classical Greek and Roman times as digestive stimulants and medicines, a twin use that continues to this day.

Black mustard was prized for its greater heat, more pungent flavour and higher amounts of volatile oil. It had the problem, however, of being unusually tall (up to 3m or 12ft high) and of shedding its seeds too readily at harvest time – appropriate in a weed but less so in a cultivated crop. These shortcomings have reduced black mustard's appeal in today's world of mechanised harvesting, and more moderate brown mustards from the East have taken its place in most commercial blends.

White mustard has retained a bitter, somewhat acrid taste that has always been appreciated by the English. Its strong preservative qualities, which prevent moulds and stop bacterial growth, have made it a useful pickling spice and antimicrobial.

It was found long ago that the aromatic oils of mustard are quiescent in the dry state as seeds or powder, which allowed it to be stored without losing strength. Until about 1720 English mustard was pounded with flour in a quern and mixed with wine vinegar; it was sold as mustard balls. Then a Mrs Clements of Durham discovered a replicable method of milling mustard seeds into a powder, presented this to the king, and made her mustard famous. A contemporary was impressed that 'we have it [mustard flour] always fresh, and full of brisk Spirits'.

We now know that adding cold or lukewarm water to mustard powder activates an enzyme that produces a sulphur compound with a pungent mustard smell and 'bite'. This reaction takes about 10 to 15 minutes. Mixing with hot water or vinegar deactivates the enzyme, however, yielding a mild but bitter-tasting mustard. These biochemical changes explain why flour mustard is made with tepid water just before a meal is served.

A significant innovation by the leading English mustard maker, Colman's of Norwich, in 1907 was ready-made English mustard, then sold in a stone jar and now in a tin or plastic tube. Powder is less seen on tables now as people prefer the immediacy of ready-made.

Dijon mustard is flavoured with pepper and verjuice (from unripe grapes), while American mustard is from mild brown seeds, made yellow with turmeric for hot dogs.

Use mustard for...

Mustard and pepper, our standard western condiments, are both hot but have different kinds of heat. While pepper works on the throat and upper digestive tract, mustard's heat is diffusing, and quickly spreads around the body.

This underlies the usefulness of mustard baths and foot baths – for patients with a cold headache Julie will sometimes suggest a mustard foot bath. Foot baths bring

In short, whenever a strong stimulating medicine is wanted to act upon the nervous system, without exciting much heat, there is none preferable to mustard seed.
– Meyrick (1789)

... the wonderfully deep-penetrating, rubefacient, decongesting, and pain-relieving benefits of this herbal poultice.
– Green (2000)

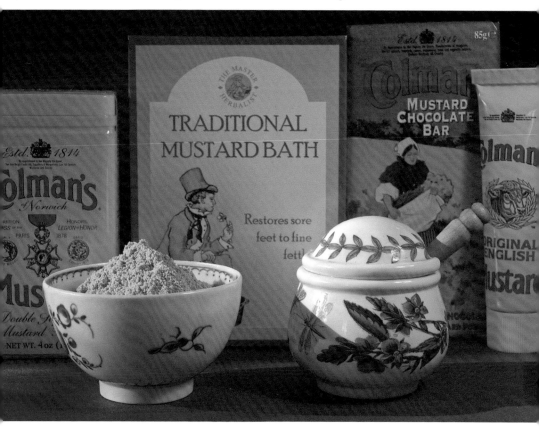

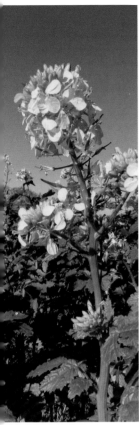
Mustard flower

excellent relief for tired feet or a chill, and improve the circulation.

An old country remedy was to put a little mustard powder in the socks to ease tired feet. And the most succinct remedy we found in our local record office was for treating chilblains: 'To prevent chilblains: Wash the feet with flour of mustard.'

Mustard poultices and plasters are old treatments for the chest. This was routine for whooping-cough in children before antibiotics. As a counter-irritant, mustard poultices draw the blood actively to the skin, making it go reddish, the sudden local heat working on underlying cold conditions.

Chest poultices relieve congestion and help expectorate mucus and dry coughs, and relieve conditions like bronchitis. The poultice should be thick enough to keep the mustard from direct contact with the skin.

Mustard powder mixed with a carrier oil, eg sunflower or almond oil, and warmed, can be massaged on sore joints and tired muscles, again with provisos for those with sensitive skin. But oil of mustard – the distilled essential oil – is too caustic for any skin.

Mustard grows everywhere, in cultivation and wild, and is cheap, if not free. The young, fresh shoots are a standby or famine food, with mustard greens especially popular in China and Japan. Mustard and cress (*Lepidium sativum*) remains a supermarket salad and sandwich, just as it was in Victorian times.

Mustard poultice
- chills
- warms and revitalises or reinvogorates the whole body

Mustard foot bath
- after a long walk
- hot feet
- tired feet
- aching legs & feet
- head cold

In terms of quantity there is more mustard used throughout the world than any other flavouring or spice, except pepper.
– Howes (1973)

Mustard poultice
Start with a handful of **mustard powder** and the same amount of a dilutent such as cornflour (cornstarch). Mix mustard powder with a little *warm* **water** to make a paste; mix cornflour with *hot* water into a paste. Combine the pastes. Place a thin cloth on the skin and spread the poultice mixture thickly on it.

Leave the poultice on for up to half an hour on normal skin, for reddening to occur but not blistering; for sensitive skins leave on for much less time, say 5 minutes. Pay close attention to the skin's reaction.

Mustard foot bath
Find a basin large enough to put your feet in comfortably. Mix 2 tablespoonfuls of **mustard powder** with about 10 cups of **hot water** in the basin. As soon as the water has cooled enough to be comfortable, put your feet in and soak them for 20 minutes while you relax.

Nutmeg & mace *Myristica fragrans*

Of all the spices 'from the East', none were more exotic or mysterious than nutmeg and mace. Their trade was as high-risk and profitable as the hard drugs of today, but much of their claimed effectiveness, as in treating plague or as an aphrodisiac, was self-deluding. They had more mundane medicinal value for nervous and digestive disorders, and were rightly valued as cooking spices. Today, nutmeg is an excellent herbal sedative.

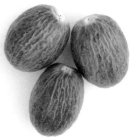

Myristicaceae
Myristica family
(Magnolia order)

Description: Maritime tropical evergreen trees, 7–10m (22–33ft) tall, with small oval leaves, yellow flowers and fruit, giving mace and nutmeg.

Distribution: Native to the Moluccas, now grown in West Indies, India, Sri Lanka, Indonesia and Australia.

Parts used: Unusually, one tree with two different spices; nutmeg powder is often taken in capsule form. In Chinese medicine nutmeg is *rou dou kou*.

You wouldn't expect nutmeg to be so beautiful. The tree is a tropical evergreen of medium height, with glossy dark-green leaves. Its fruit is like a golden, palm-size lemon, with yellow flesh. When ripe, the fruit cuts open to reveal the nut.

A coral red, moist, hand-like aril, the mace, encloses and feeds a striated, darker single nut, the nutmeg. Sadly, both lose their freshness within a day of picking and drying, the mace turning dull orange and the nutmeg, now removed from its shell, becoming a mediocre mid-brown.

To European eyes the hard brown nutmegs or blades of orangey mace were not as visually attractive as cinnamon bark, as intriguing as cloves or pungent like pepper. So why did nutmeg command high prices?

Nutmeg was the ultimate mystery spice in medieval western Europe. It came 'from the East', said Arab traders; perpetuating such exotic vagueness was a tactic in maintaining a valuable monopoly. The supply was small, secret and defendable, the demand for the product insatiable – conditions for the perfect monopoly, as the Arabs, Venetians, Portuguese, Dutch and English in turn knew.

The actual source of all this clamour, the spice islands, were remote indeed – six small volcanic islands in the Banda group of the Moluccas, a thousand kilometres north of Australia. One island, Run, had precisely the balance of soil and microclimate that suited nutmeg's exacting demands. Its trees gave several harvests a year, yielded for seventy years and needed little tending.

Run became so precious that in 1667 the Dutch traded

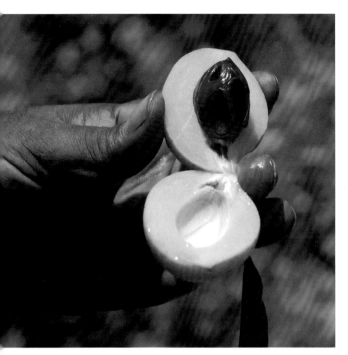

Use nutmeg and mace for...

Both mace and nutmeg yield rich volatile oils, chiefly myristicin and elemicin, which have narcotic qualities, but only in very large quantities. In small amounts nutmeg and mace give up intensive flavours to cooked food, mace being strong and pungent, nutmeg sweet and warming. There is little evidence, though, as is often supposed, that nutmeg was used for preserving rank meat: there were other, local, strong and inexpensive herbs for that.

Nor was there was any proof for nutmeg's efficacy as a remedy for the plague, but it was sold at high prices to the desperate. It had more success in checking the all-too-common and sometimes fatal 'bloody flux', a virulent dysentery.

Nutmeg was more ordinarily a treatment for diarrhoea, vomiting, colic and fevers – the druggists' 'aromatic powder', mixed from nutmeg, cinnamon, ginger and cardamom, being a popular spice nostrum. It was also used as an anti-inflammatory for the skin and for rheumatic conditions.

Was nutmeg an aphrodisiac? High price and exclusivity, along with intense aroma, go with the territory, but there is little actual direct evidence of such use in western herbal traditions. At some point, the old phrase about nutmeg became true: 'a medicine in the East, a condiment in the West'. Hence Indian Ayurveda

... it has been found by Experience, that the frequent and excessive use, both of the Nuts and Bark, occasions Sleepy Diseases, for they are very Narcotick.
– Pechey (1707)

Nutmeg is found by experience to be a very useful herb in the treatment of insomnia, and if used in doses of 6–7g daily has no real adverse effects. It would appear that true poisonings have only occurred when there are much higher doses of at least 20g.
– Herbert (2008)

their island of New Amsterdam for it, thereby gifting Manhattan to the English. It must be the deal of that century, a telling statement of the lure of nutmeg.

Trading profits for nutmeg could be astounding and worth huge risks: while Shakespeare was writing and performing his plays at the Globe theatre in Southwark, traders in the City were selling five kilos (10.5lb) of nutmeg for £2 10s. This was a 600-fold profit, as the same bag cost less than a penny in Run – a comparable mark-up to that of today's illegal heroin or cocaine trade.

readily prescribes nutmeg for male sexual problems and for the female menstrual cycle.

A current use of nutmeg, in East and West, is as a tonic for insomnia. Julie and other herbalists have found nutmeg to be especially valuable for the kind of insomnia where you wake in the middle of the night and are unable to go back to sleep.

Nutmeg is slow acting but long lasting. It has a 12-hour cycle, acting after four hours but continuing for eight more. A patient wanting to sleep at 10pm would take the capsules at 6pm and expect to wake as normal after 6am.

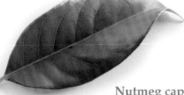

Nutmeg does not suit everybody, though it works well for most people. If you take too much for you, it can make you feel spacey – be cautious if you are driving or operating machinery. The right dose will just make you feel delightfully relaxed, and a low dose is wonderful for anxiety.

Is nutmeg a poison? Not on the above regime. There are few authenticated cases of poisoning, and only for very high doses. And an hallucinogen? Nutmeg is sometimes compared with the rave drug Ecstasy, and indeed is chemically similar. But only huge amounts of nutmeg – difficult to hold down in the stomach – give the drug effect. This is an undeserved abuse of Meyrick's (1789) 'moderately warm and grateful spice'.

Nutmeg capsules

Because nutmeg has such a strong flavour, it is difficult to take enough for insomnia as a spice in food, and making your own capsules (or buying them from a herbalist) is your best option.

Freshly grate **nutmeg** and use the powder to fill **empty capsules** (available from herbal suppliers).

Dose: the dosage of nutmeg is very person-specific. For insomnia, start with one capsule, and increase by one capsule a night until a good sleep pattern emerges: 2 or 3 is enough for most people but you may need up to 8 or even 10 capsules a night (if it isn't working at that dose, it isn't the herb for you). Usually the nutmeg can be discontinued after the pattern of insomnia has been broken.

A lower dose, usually just one capsule, can be used as a daytime remedy for anxiety.

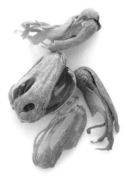

Oats *Avena sativa*

Oats is a major food crop of northern latitudes, where wheat and barley struggle to mature. Porridge, gruel, groats, oatmeal cakes and haggis are among its nutritious forms, while medicinally the unripened tops and straw yield a warming restorative tonic for the nervous system, for improving blood cholesterol balance and for certain skin problems.

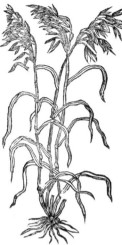

Oats, from Parkinson's *Theatrum Botanicum* (1640)

Graminae (Poaceae) Grass family

Description: Slender annual cereal, with husked drooping fruit, the tops cropped medicinally when still green and milky, and the grain harvested when ripe for food production.

Distribution: Cultivated mainly in northern latitudes, in moist, temperate and cool climates.

Related species: Wild oat (*A. fatua*) and others from southern Europe and East Asia are distant progenitors of the cultivated form.

Parts used: Green immature tops, straw, ripe grain.

Oats was a latecomer among the world's major cereals, with all those wild oats sowing themselves and refusing to settle down. It was not until about 1000 BC that cultivators in central and southern Europe bred a strain of oats that could be reliably harvested. The Greeks and Romans dismissed oats as barbarian food, although the Romans brought it to Britain to feed their horses and encouraged oats-growing in Wales and Scotland.

Oats and horses enjoyed a linked working history in agriculture and in warfare until the twentieth century. Horses, fed on oats pulled trailers and ploughs, and also wheeled guns. As horses were replaced by machines, oats growing diminished – although porridge never lost its primacy in Scotland – but was revived by the emergence of muesli, with oats as its cereal base, and porridge as a low glycaemic index food. British stores now feature attractively packaged oatcakes, sometimes flavoured with ginger, cranberries and other non-traditional tastes.

If oats is stamina food for horses, it is equally nutritious for people. An old Irish saying went: 'Rye bread will do you good, / Barley bread will do you no harm, / Wheat bread will sweeten your blood, / Oat bread will strengthen your arm.' Oats is low in the gluten that binds bread together, so oat bread is necessarily mixed with wheat or other flour. Emigrants from Scotland to North America in the nineteenth century would take such oat loaves to sustain them on the Atlantic voyage, along with their ever-present oatcakes.

The Scots of course will always be associated with porridge, the staple diet for much of the national history. In 1785, it was 'halesome parritch, chief of Scotia's food', according to Robert Burns. In 1771, another poet, Robert Fergusson, wrote: 'On sicken food has mony a doughty deed / by Caledonia's ancestors been done.'

Not all the English disparaged oats as much as Samuel Johnson famously did ('a grain, which in England is generally given to horses, but in Scotland supports the people'): in 1949, the English herbalist Mrs Leyel noted that 'oats as a brain food are extremely valuable, and the Scot who lives on porridge can work harder and longer mentally than most races'.

This is well said, though hard to prove, but consider this: their oats diet enabled the Scots to flourish in damp, cold conditions and poor soils, survive clan rivalry, war with and occupation by the English, plague and enforced emigration – and yet never suffer harvest failure on a scale to match that of the Irish potato famine. Enlightenment Edinburgh was 'the Venice of the north', plus oats.

Use oats for...

Fergusson had succinctly labelled oats 'sicken food'. It is one of oats' great blessings that it makes such a ready source of nutrition in illness and convalescence, especially for 'nervous' and deficiency conditions; additionally, having insignificant gluten, oats is excellent recuperation fare for those with wheat intolerance.

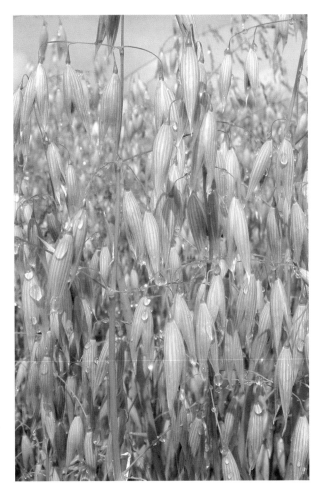

Oats products are easily made and digested, conveying protein, more fat than any other cereal, vitamins (including the B group), minerals (including calcium, iron, zinc and silicon), saponins and digestible fibre. Oats starch readily gelatinises and creams on cooking – which is why you need to stir your porridge as it simmers or it will stick to the pan!

Children and the sick who find taking the more solid porridge difficult may tolerate a watery oats gruel. This was a sickroom standby for centuries, in forms such as pottages, broths and oats ale that are mostly ignored today. Two Scots variations were brose, made from oatmeal on which boiling water was poured, and

When Corn is dear, poor People live chiefly on Water-gruel [oats]: And it is indeed, very proper Diet for Sick and Well, and yields a good nourishment. ... Our Physicians scarce order any Diet but Water-Gruel in Acute Diseases.
– Pechey (1707)

the resulting gruel eaten with milk; and sowans or sowins, made from oats husks, infused in water for a week (that is, became sour) and then boiled down to form a nutritious jelly.

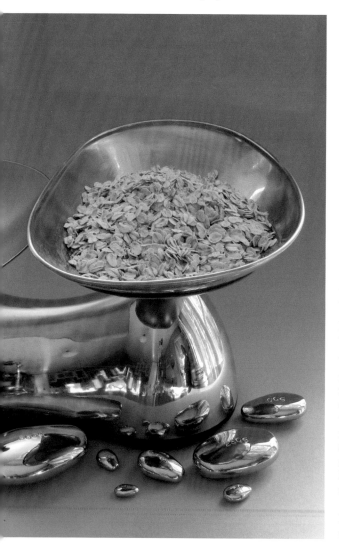

Oats has a traditional external use as an anti-inflammatory for itchy skin conditions, including eczema and shingles. Uncooked oatmeal can be added to the bath, either via a strained decoction or directly through soaking a gauze bag containing the meal in the water. Abbé Kneipp in late nineteenth-century France added oats to baths for skin problems, and arthritic, rheumatic and liver conditions.

In 1692, Thomas Tryon wrote of using oats in 'an excellent poultice' for 'Burns, Scalded Limbs, Boyls, Fellons, Tumers … Inflammations, Contuzions, or Bruizes'. He added ground oatmeal to 'good water', sugar and chopped dandelion, boiled them together and applied the poultice to the affected part.

Earlier, in 1602, Sir Hugh Plat championed a simple chilblain remedy in which oats boiled in water were put in a bowl covered by a double cloth, the hands (or feet) being held 'within the Oats as hot as you may well suffer them'.

Looking at oats internally, modern research establishes that eating it regularly helps reduce blood cholesterol levels, lowering the 'bad' LDL cholesterol quickly and raising the 'good' HDL type more slowly. This action makes oats a dietary ally in combating coronary heart disease and a preventative measure against colon cancer.

Modern American herbalism makes extensive use of immature

green oats flowers, known as 'oatseed' and stems, or 'oatstraw', in a milky tonic or tincture that is sweet and nutritious, for the conditions already described. Oat milk is readily made (we use rolled oats as easier to source) or is sold in modern supermarkets; we advocate its use in cooking as a dairy replacement.

In the early twentieth century proponents had been keen to claim that medicinal use of oatseed and oatstraw assisted withdrawal from addictions such as tobacco and alcohol. These claims are not recognised by orthodox medicine. But that does not mean oats has been discredited. Far from it, for its powerful supportive effect to both mind and body in conditions of stress and exhaustion – facts of contemporary life for many of us – has brought oats a wider purpose and value than ever before.

... when the [oat] ears are just beginning to form, when it is juicy and breaking into flower, this green grass is at its richest in avenin, which is unsurpassed as a nutrient for the cells of the nervous system.
– Dr Vogel (1952)

If you're worried about blood cholesterol, there hardly seems a better food pharmaceutical than oats.
– Carper (1989)

Oat bath

Put a cup of **oatmeal** in a square of muslin or a cloth handkerchief, or an old sock. Hang the bag or sock from the hot tap while you run a bath, or place it in the tub under the hot running water.

Once the bath has run, you can use the bag like a sponge to rub over your skin, releasing the soothing oat milk. Afterwards, throw away the oats and wash the cloth for using next time.

Oat milk

Soak 1 cup rolled **oats** in 5 cups **water** overnight.
Place in a blender and blend until smooth.
It can be used as is, or strained if you prefer. You might like to add a teaspoon of **vanilla** extract.

Athol brose

A modern luxury version of a traditional sweet. A non-alcoholic alternative might substitute apple juice for the whisky.

Toast 1 cup **rolled oats** in a cast iron or non-stick pan, using a medium heat until it gently browns (do not allow to burn). Mix 2 tablespoons **runny honey,** 2 tablespoons **whisky** and 1 teaspoonful **vanilla** extract in a bowl. Whip 300ml **double cream** or whipping cream until it feels light, and add to the bowl. Add the crunchy oatmeal just before serving and fold gently into the cream mixture. Spoon into two tall glasses.

For an even more luxurious treat, layer the oat and cream mixture with blueberries, raspberries or sliced strawberries.

Oat bath
• itchy skin
• eczema
• rashes

Oat milk
• dairy substitute

Athol brose
• aphrodisiac
• energising
• lifts the spirits

Olive *Olea europaea*

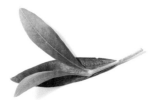

**Oleaceae
Olive family**

Description: A characteristic public and cultivated evergreen tree of the Mediterranean, to 10m (30ft) tall – very old individuals can be as wide and become convoluted; grey–green trunk and lanceolate, leathery leaves, small greeny-white flowers and plentiful fruit, green at first and often ripening to black or white, of many varieties.

Distribution: Probably native to E Mediterranean and the Fertile Crescent, now widespread in the Mediterranean and similar climatic zones around the world. Hardy in occasional frost and prefers semi-arid conditions (hence not in tropics or deserts).

Related species: Wild olive (*O. europaea* subsp. *oleaster*) may be the progenitor of the cultivated olive; it is smaller, with some spines and bears a smaller, more astringent fruit.

Parts used: Oil, leaves, fruit.

The olive is one of the oldest of the Old World trees, with a range of traditional medicinal applications in addition to the familiar use of olive oil for cooking and black or green olives for eating. The leaves have been discovered (or, more accurately, rediscovered) to be valuable medicinally in their own right.

Plant historians believe that the olive tree was domesticated in the Fertile Crescent of the Tigris–Euphrates valley some 10,000 years ago, finding a ready and permanent home around the Mediterranean coast in succeeding millennia. With the date palm, fig and grape, olive is among the earliest of mankind's fruit crops.

These early olives were small, bitter and astringent, like the wild olive of today, and more palatable as an expressed oil than as an esculent fruit. In the literature of classical Greece and Rome it is the oil that is the object of desire – the Latin for 'olive' is practically the same word as the generic 'oil'.

In Rome, as in Greece and Egypt earlier, olive oil was the anointing oil of choice and the means of domestic lighting, in addition to its essential role in cooking. Olive oil, along with availability of hot water, enabled a culture of personal cleanliness in the great Mediterranean civilisations.

The Romans knew that what benefited the skin also worked

for the liver, and vice versa, swallowing an olive oil purge to help eliminate gallstones as well as ease constipation. These ancient discoveries remain valid.

An old Roman health cliché summed up: 'wine within and oil without'. The health benefits of the Mediterranean diet are now well known, and traditionally prepared pure olive oil is an integral part of that diet and way of life.

The best kind of olive oil both for our taste buds and our kitchen medicine is organic, cold pressed and extra virgin. This is taken from the first pressing, has an acidity of under 1% and retains the active principles of the fruit (the bitter principle, oleuropein, is largely removed in the spinning process). There is no heating, filtering or chemical extraction.

These exacting standards actually reproduce those of the old-fashioned olive grower of previous centuries who was too poor to be anything other than organic and had only a water-driven millstone to crush his olive harvest.

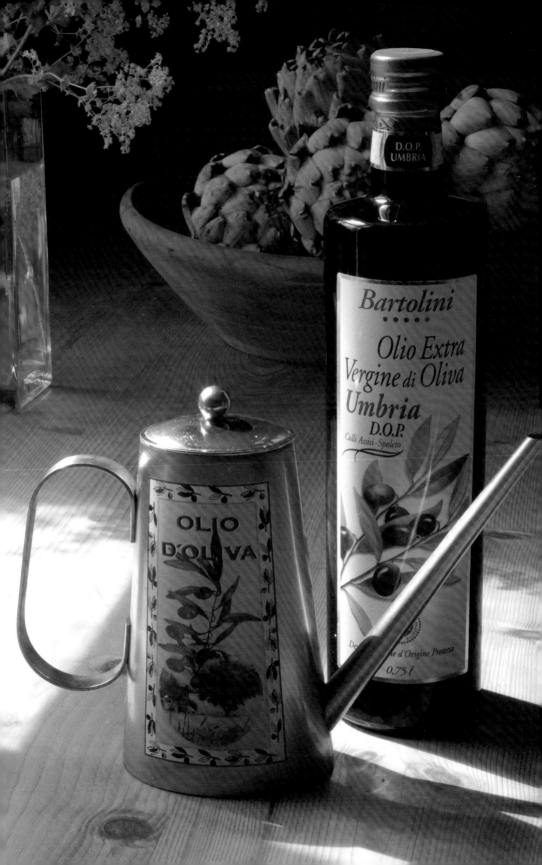

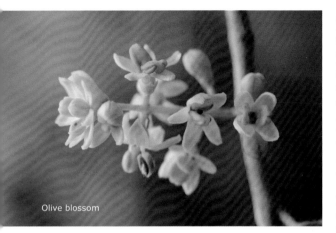
Olive blossom

gastric secretions and allays the pain of gastric and peptic ulcers. The warming and moderately laxative nature of the oil also stimulates the sphincters in the digestive system, meaning that stagnant food is moved along. A spoonful of olive oil (tea or tablespoon size, at your discretion) taken first thing in the morning is a Greek and Roman remedy for constipation that still works today.

Modern life can be quite hard on the liver. Fatty and processed foods, anger and emotional strain, alcohol and coffee all take their toll. The liver has to deal with toxins – environmental pollution, pesticides on food, excess hormones, household chemicals, poisonous emotions – and neutralise them to minimise harm to us. If you're feeling sluggish, tired or muddle-headed, chances are your liver would benefit from the gentle liver cleanse drink on the next page, which uses olive oil to stimulate the flow of bile.

Olive leaves also have remarkable healing benefits, and can be taken as a tea to lower blood sugar levels and improve the circulation. Olive leaf's astringency is key, with its antiviral, antibiotic, antifungal and antiparasitic benefits. It helps destroy or neutralise over a hundred disease-causing micro-organisms, it has been claimed, including the common cold, malaria and candida. If you have access to olive leaves, try making an infusion for yourself.

A superior oil
Olive oil is unusual, and superior, among vegetable oils for its high ratio of unsaturated fatty acids (65–85% by volume of monounsaturated oleic acid and 7–15% of di-unsaturated linoleic acid), in a highly beneficial combination for the heart; vitamin E and antioxidants are among the 1–2% of the residual products.

Evidence suggests that using olive oil as a regular part of the diet, in salads and as a cooking oil, is more protective of heart health than saturated and polyunsaturated fats. The antioxidants in the oil help the body fight off cancers and circulatory dysfunction. Drinking small amounts of the oil has been specifically linked to prevention of atherosclerosis.

Use olives for…

Olive oil is stable, warming and nutritive; it excludes air, does not dry out or go rancid; it flows at room temperature; and it softens and coats the surfaces it encounters. In the nineteenth century the oil was used as a delicate grease for watches and clocks. Olive oil is wonderful for the skin, and is our favourite oil for making ointments and infusing with herbs.

The oil can also be used on the hair as a scalp rub and to combat dandruff. It is a good rub for rheumatism, and a reasonable (though stickier) massage oil if almond oil is not available. Olive oil soaps have been called 'a Mediterranean diet for the skin'.

The oil's soothing effects function similarly internally by adding a thin protective coating to the stomach and intestinal walls. This demulcent property reduces

Gentle liver cleanse

This drink is most effective taken first thing in the morning, at least half an hour before eating, but can be drunk any time of day.

Put in a blender: a big glassful of **apple juice** – fresh squeezed is best, but packaged is fine. Add the **juice of a lemon** or lime, freshly squeezed. (If you prefer, you can use all fresh-squeezed citrus juices.) Add a clove of **garlic**, a chunk of **fresh ginger**, 1 tablespoon of **extra virgin olive oil**, and blend well. The lemon and other juices emulsify the oil and the finished drink is actually very pleasant – foamy and gingery.

If you want to, you can dilute the mixture to taste with spring water. Drink slowly, holding each mouthful for a moment before swallowing. Follow about 15 minutes later with a cup of herb tea, such as ginger, peppermint or fennel.

The first few times you take this drink, it may make you feel a little queasy. This means it is working and is a sign you really need it. Drink less or dilute it with water if the feeling is too strong, and follow with a cup of fresh ginger tea.

This drink will give you garlicky breath, so try to do it on days when you don't have to be too close to people, or chew some fresh parsley or cardamom pods to help clear the garlic smell. Take 2 or 3 times a week, or as often as you feel in need of it.

Gentle liver cleanse
- tiredness
- hangovers
- feeling sluggish
- muddle-headedness
- tired eyes
- hormone imbalances
- overindulgence

The oil lubricates, softens, nourishes, and unkinks.
– Wood (2008)

We do well to treasure a fruit which has nourished so many so well and for so long (at least since 1700 years BC) and seems to have helped protect them from degenerative disease.
– Barker (2001)

Infused oil

To make an infused oil, put the **herb** of your choice in a jar, then fill with **olive oil** and place on a sunny windowsill for up to a month. Strain and bottle. A sprig or two of the herb can be added to the bottle for decoration. If you are using the oil for cooking, it can be diluted to taste with more oil.

Try infusing garlic, rosemary, chillies, thyme or mustard. The oil can be easily made into an ointment by heating it with beeswax: use 1 part wax to 4 parts oil by weight.

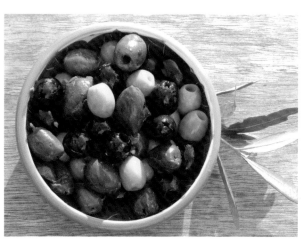

Onion *Allium cepa*

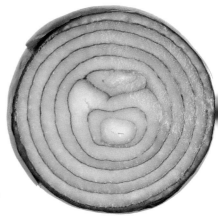

Onions are much better known these days in cooking and gardening terms than as a standby home medicine. That is unfortunate, and we'd like to make a case for the defence.

**Liliaceae
Lily family**

Description: Biennial or perennial, reaching 1m (36in) and more in some forms; usually 4–6 cylindrical, hollow green leaves; green–white, small flowers, in umbels or bulbils; the swollen, fleshy single or multiple root is the 'onion'.

Distribution: Probably originates in the Middle East or central Asia, but domesticated so long that its ancestry is problematic; widespread in temperate and subtropical areas worldwide.

Related species: *Allium cepa* can be subdivided three ways: *Cepas* proper, which have single, round bulbs; *Proliferums*, the tree onions; and *Aggregatums*, the shallots. Other familiar *Alliums* include garlic (*A. sativum*), leeks (*A. porrum*) and scallions (*A. fistulosum*).

Parts used: Fresh bulb, juice, stems in some species (eg spring onions, leeks).

The onion is not an obvious 'lily of the field', in the Biblical phrase, but it is an economically important member of the lily family. There are around 500 alliums, linked by their 'biting' sulphur compounds, more apparent in some onion species, especially garlic, less so in leeks, chives, shallots or scallions.

The ancient Egyptians regarded the onion as a symbol of the layers of eternity. White and mild-tasting onions were the staple of the labourers who built the Pyramids, along with bread and beer. The Greek historian Herodotus records with some disbelief that the pharaohs used 1600 talents of silver to pay for onions and radishes.

Onions also accompanied the dead, with dried plants discovered with many prominent mummies. Egyptian priests, though, like today's Brahmin priests in India, were not allowed to eat onions; the results were too stimulating.

In 1699 John Evelyn echoed this implicit class approach to onion:

'… an honest laborious Countryman, with good Bread, Salt, and a little Parsley, will make a contented meal with a roasted Onion'. In 1825 the French gastronome Brillat-Savarin could state that 'the onion is the truffle of the poor'.

Garden onions will dry out to some nine-tenths of their fresh weight, which makes them notably easy to store and transport. They keep in a cool kitchen for weeks if uncut, though if you store them sliced in the fridge add some bicarbonate of soda for the smell.

The excellent natural wrapping of an onion keeps the volatile oils inactive but, as everybody knows, once you cut the skin and chop an onion a chemical reaction occurs that can lead to eye irritation with copious tears and the characteristic sharp, acrid aroma.

What makes the onion special as a food is that continued heating will caramelise the onion flesh, turning its starches to sugars, neutralising the 'bite' and adding 'umami'.

It can almost be claimed that onions are a good base for any hot meal, sweetening and deepening taste and improving satiety. The long domestic history suggests that most civilisations would agree. Presently some 64 million tonnes are produced annually, and onion is the second most popular horticultural crop after tomatoes.

The Libyans are now the biggest onion consumers, at over 65lb (28kg) per person per year, but India, China and the US are not far behind. The cropped area worldwide is increasing, while onions remain an easy homegrown crop. Alliums have colourful, sculptural flowers and make striking garden plants, with the added benefit of being good in companion planting schemes.

This expansion in culinary and horticultural applications does, however, seem to have been at the expense of the traditional reputation of onion as a medicinal plant. This use is still (just) within oral tradition, and we hope we can reinforce it here. It would be sad if onions – like leeks and chives, say – were only known as food.

Onion in verse
For this is every cook's opinion, /
No savoury dish without an onion./
But lest your kissing should be spoiled, /
Your onions must be fully boiled.
– Swift (c. 1720)

If envious age relax the nuptial knot, /
Thy food be scallions and thy feast shallot.
– Martial (c. AD 100)

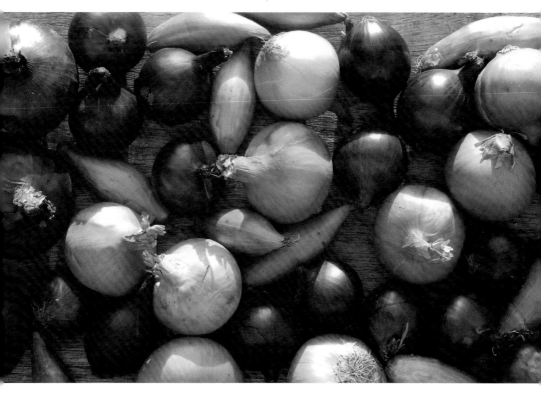

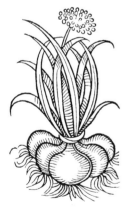

A medieval image of an onion

Use onions for...

Cutting and eating raw onion must be one of the easiest and oldest of herbal remedies. In 1952, in Horseheath, Cambridgeshire, a local saying was recorded: 'If an onion is eaten every morning before breakfast, all the doctors might ride on one horse.'

Onion is highly versatile as a domestic remedy: the juice can be used; the bulb can be made into a gruel or a thicker soup; it can be macerated in water or milk, and drunk or used as a poultice; it can be mixed with honey as a syrup and with wine or spirits as a tincture; it can be pickled or dried.

By comparing oral records from the 1920s and 1990s mainly in East Anglia, herbal historian Gabrielle Hatfield has shown how onions are just within memory in home treatment of respiratory ailments.

Onion is warming and drawing for mucus, pus and poisons; it is antimicrobial and antispasmodic in effect. It was an old remedy for cutting mucus embedded in the lungs and helping to eliminate it; traditionally it was used to soothe asthma, especially as a poultice placed on the chest.

American herbalist Richo Cech describes vividly how he eased his small child's winter breathing difficulties by frying an onion in olive oil, stirring in a cup of vinegar and some handfuls of cornmeal. He put the resulting stiff paste onto a diaper (nappy), about an inch thick, tucking the ends under the child's armpits, and then covering the diaper with a plastic bag, towel and blanket. The child recovered within a day.

Onion is antiseptic and can be used as such in emergencies. Anecdotal reports suggest that Russian soldiers in the Second World War applied onions to battle wounds, and in the American Civil War General Ulysses S. Grant used onion juice as an antiseptic. Onion is a traditional remedy for treating ear infections, including 'glue ear', both as a small poultice and as juice applied to the ear.

Further back in time, onion was a plague and cholera treatment, and used against internal worms. It was long believed to be effective for 'cancerous complaints'. Onion was also taken for 'the nerves', for exhaustion and to increase appetite. It was used to prolong and deepen sleep, and to clear the air passages.

Not surprisingly in a more literal age, being all skin itself, onion was employed in many skin disorders. It was and still is good for treating wasp stings. A letter to an early nineteenth-century English newspaper recorded that 'I have seen it tried with the smallest scallion from a sallad. The effect is instantaneous in curing the pain.'

It was used on fresh burns, and offered pain relief, a fact known

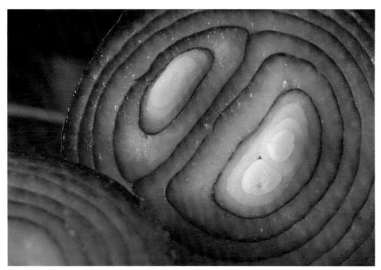

[An onion] *poultice is simply vegetable material, whole or mashed, which is layered or spread on the skin. ... The hot poultice increases circulation, while the cold poultice reduces inflammation.*
– Cech (2000)

[On making a red onion poultice for skin cancer] *Slice it, & braize it in a marble mortar, taking great care that no metal of any sort comes near it.*
– Sophia Baillie (1819)

by schoolboys about to be caned. Onion also served as a hair restorer, to remove blemishes and acne, and draw splinters; its outer skin could be an emergency plaster. It was popularly used to treat water retention (oedema); it eased problems of urine retention, and added to perspiration. It also increased blood circulation and boosted the iron content of the blood in cases of anaemia.

Research has shown that onion lowers blood cholesterol and blood sugars, giving it a role in easing blood pressure and preventing blood clots. Onion is also a dietary support in type-2 diabetes.

Onion poultice

Onion is versatile enough to make successful poultices cooked or raw, cold or warm, from fresh or using onion powder or flakes. At the most basic, cut an onion and apply wet side to a bite or swelling and cover with a cloth. Cutting releases the healing alkaloids, and covering gives the onion a chance to draw out the poison, heat or inflammation.

If you have more time, peel the onion and chop it into small pieces, either raw or cooked with olive oil, as you prefer. Then place the pieces in the centre of a square of fabric, like a T-shirt or flannel, and roll the ends over to make a packet. Attach the sides with safety pins, if to hand. If the mixture is too mushy, add cornflour or other powder. Then apply to the skin and keep it there. Check every few minutes for any adverse reactions, such as skin irritation, in which case stop.

Onion poultice
- draws poison, heat, stings, splinters
- breaks up congestion of colds and 'flu as a chest poultice
- improves sluggish circulation
- treatment for asthma

Orange

Bitter or Seville orange *Citrus aurantium* var. *amara;* **Sweet orange** *Citrus aurantium* var. *dulcis*

Rutaceae
Rue family

Description: Small tree, to 10m (33ft) tall and 6m (20ft) wide; rough, spiny branches and green, shiny, oval leaves; large, fragrant white flowers; circular fruits with orange aromatic rind and fleshy, acidic pulp.

Distribution: The citrus family was native to SE Asia and S China, spreading westwards over the last three millennia; bitter oranges as such are grown mostly in Spain. Predominantly commercial cultivation in groves, especially near sea coast, away from frost.

Related species: Sweet orange (*C. aurantium* var. *dulcis, C. sinensis*); bergamot orange (*C. aurantium* var. *bergamia*); lemon (*C. limon*); lime (*C. aurantiifolia*); mandarin, tangerine, satsuma (*C. reticulata*); grapefruit (*C. paradisi*).

Parts used: Bitter orange peel, bergamot oil (from bergamot orange); leaves (petitgrain oil); flowers (neroli oil, orange flower water); whole fruit; sweet orange fruit used mainly for juice and eaten fresh.

Citrus growers and breeders should be botanical heroes for the wonderfully diverse products they have given us. There is much more to oranges than their juice or marmalade, with varied medicinal applications.

The citruses originated in China or Southeast Asia and began moving to the west via conquest and trade at least three millennia ago, probably the first fruit family to make this journey. Pips of citron (*Citrus medica*), a precursor of modern oranges, found in Cyprus have been dated to 1200 BC. The name 'orange' itself hints at an exotic past: it comes via Arabic from Sanskrit *nagarunga*, 'the fruit elephants like'.

Sweet orange is a familiar domestic fruit everywhere, and orange juice is the cold breakfast drink of choice (though not ours: we find it mixes badly with milk and tea or coffee at the same meal). Brazil and the United States dominate the world market in growing and processing oranges into FCOJ, or frozen concentrate orange juice, the means by which a subtropical fruit can be served all year round worldwide.

Such juice is a good source of vitamin C, but comes with many chemical additions. The best orange juice is no doubt that which you squeeze for yourself from fresh oranges that you know are organically grown.

By comparison, the bitter or Seville orange, the most medicinal of the citrus family, has a tiny food market. Much of the crop is exported to Britain for commercial marmalade; in January and February each year British cooks hunt out the season's supply of Sevilles for a home-made version.

The bitterness of the marmalade oranges is tempered, though not overwhelmed, by plentiful sugar, and the rind that carries the embedded oil glands is retained, whether 'thin cut' or 'thick'. Growers are not permitted to wax Seville skins (sweet orange skins are not as lucky), so it is safe to use them in your marmalade, in your infusions and other preparations.

Bitter oranges form the woodstock for grafting other orange varieties. They also have a role in the perfumery industry, yielding three different essential oils, all also used medicinally.

Use orange for...

Neroli is the oil of orange flowers, an expensive but fantastic fragrance that is uplifting, sedative and antidepressant. Physically, it is an antiseptic and can calm the stomach. Use in the bath or as a massage oil, with a neutral carrier like almond oil. Parkinson (1640) recommended an orange flower ointment 'to anoint the stomacke to help the cough, and to expectorate the cold, raw flegme'.

Orange flower water, a by-product of neroli distillation, scents desserts and pastries. It was the Victorian lady's standby for every emergency, and also gentle enough to relieve baby colic.

Bergamot orange originated in early seventeenth-century Bergamo, in north Italy, and is inedible; the rind, however, is pressed for **bergamot oil**, an antibacterial used to treat shingles and urinary tract infections, especially in women. It is the flavouring in Earl Grey tea.

Petitgrain is an essential oil processed from orange leaves. It is a gentle astringent and used on the skin; again, take in a bath or by massage with a carrier oil.

Eau-de-Cologne is the most famous herbal water, developed in eighteenth-century Germany as a facial rinse. Its original formulation was bergamot and neroli oil, with rosemary leaves, distilled in grape juice.

Orange leaves make a mild herb tea that is sedative and can raise the body temperature into a sweat, helping to break fevers. **Orange peel**, without the pith, either eaten fresh, taken in a tea, tincture or other remedy, is a digestive

The rinde of the [bitter] Orrenges are bitterer and hotter than those of Lemmons, or Citrons, and therefore doe warme a cold stomacke the more, helping to breake the winde therein, and the flegme ... the juyce is far inferior to either of them.
– Parkinson (1640)

The sour or Seville orange is the type used in medicine, the peel more than the juice or pulp ... the great use of the peel is in tincture or infusion as a stomachic.
– Hill (1812)

... [orange] promotes increased appetite and digestion, raises the blood sugar, and helps the cells plump up with water and nutrients. As a result, the skin is soft, full, velvety, and more sensitive.
– Wood (2008)

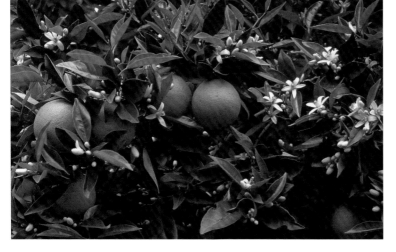

Sweet oranges, Cyprus, April

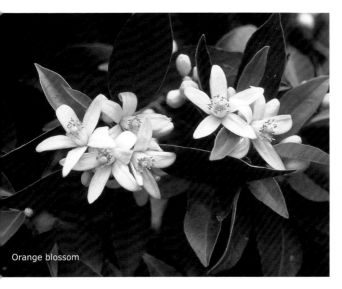
Orange blossom

stimulant that also eases flatulence and calms a stomach upset by nausea or morning sickness. It is an expectorant, loosening mucus, and a mild diuretic. Combining with orange's plentiful vitamin C, it helps fight colds and tonsillitis.

Orange fruit in Chinese herbal medicine is used both whole and unripe (*zhi shi*), and without peel and pips but ripe (*zhi ke*); these are treatments for indigestion and coughs, and the stronger *zhi shi* for shock. In western tradition, a pomander is made from a whole orange, studded with cloves and its skin rubbed with salt. It would typically be hung in a wardrobe.

Orange & cardamom bitters
- digestive bitter
- increases appetite
- improves digestion
- improves absorption

Orange and cardamom bitters

Slice 3 **bitter oranges** and put in a large jam jar with 2 tablespoons of **cardamom pods**. Pour on enough **vodka** to cover, put the lid on and leave to macerate for two or three weeks, shaking occasionally and topping up if necessary with a little more vodka. Strain and bottle. Add a little honey to taste, if desired. Take a small liqueur glassful before or after meals to improve digestion.

In 1812, John Hill made his version with brandy or wine and the skin of bitter oranges, calling it 'as good a bitter as can be made: it prevents sickness of the stomach, and is excellent to amend the appetite'.

Bitter orange and chocolate liqueur

Slice 3 **bitter oranges** and put in a large jam jar with 3 tablespoons **cocoa nibs or cocoa powder** (the nibs are best if you can get them, as the powder is harder to strain, leaving an alcoholic sludge that is too tasty to throw out) and 2 tablespoons of **cardamom pods**. Pour on enough **whisky or vodka** to cover, put the lid on and leave to macerate for two or three weeks, shaking occasionally and topping up if needed with a little more alcohol.

Strain and add **honey** to taste, then bottle. Can be served as is, but is even better mixed with some fresh **cream** before serving.

Oregano
Origanum vulgare **Wild or common oregano, Wild marjoram**

Marjoram
O. majorana, Majorana hortensis **Sweet, common or knotted marjoram**

Marjoram and oregano are close relatives that look and smell similar, and often hybridise, while their names are often confused. Just as their use in cooking can overlap, they have similar but not identical medicinal qualities. But, when it all seems too baffling, remember the pleasure that both herbs bring!

Lamiaceae (Labiatae) Mint family

The names at the top of the page encapsulate the difficulties involved in separating oregano and marjoram. Their genus is *Origanum*, but one of the two species is named oregano, also known as wild marjoram. Then, oregano is sometimes 'marjoram' in North America, and what is sold as 'oregano' may actually be a mint, thyme or verbena. In practice, too, marjorams of various kinds often hybridise with oregano in cultivation, as in the intermediate form *Origanum x applii*. Both species vary considerably in appearance and flavour according to place of origin and hours of sunshine.

This all creates a taxonomist's delight and a commercial grower's nightmare. One solution proposed is using 'oregano' as the name of a flavour rather than a plant, linking species even from different genera that contain the same 'chemical signature', namely carvacrol or thymol. It might happen one day, but the pizza makers of America

have decided already that flavour is indeed the point: what they put on their pizzas is oregano, and it tastes wonderful!

Faced by such tangles, it is good to remember the simple delight that smelling and growing these herbs brings, and their clean, tangy taste on the palate. The original Greek term 'oregano' meant 'joy of the mountain', and the wild herb was picked on joyous occasions, for wedding wreaths, and for gladsome remembrance of a life, when planted on a grave. Whether identified as marjoram or oregano, cooked with food or as home medicines, both herbs are life-affirming and uplifting.

Use oregano/marjoram for…

You may grow marjoram and oregano in the garden or kitchen to pick fresh for cooking – pot marjoram is a British favourite because it matures in most summers, though never achieving the full-on flavour of oregano from the hot European south –

Description: Oregano: robust, sprawling perennial to 60cm (24in), vertical purple/brown stems from dense rootstock, roundish green/reddish leaves, purple/pink or white flowers in clusters, with pungent scent; Marjoram: tender annual/perennial to 45cm (18in), irregular red/brown square stems, downy oval greyish leaves, tiny white/pink, 'knotted' flowers, sweet-scented, but more bitter and camphor-like on drying.

Related species: Pot marjoram or Greek oregano (*O. onites*); winter marjoram (*O. heracleoticum*); Lebanese oregano (*O. syriacum*). Commercial 'oregano' is also produced from unrelated plants.

Parts used: Leaves and flowering tops, essential oils.

but the dried young flower tops stored in cool conditions are generally stronger and preferred for medicinal use. The differences are accentuated on drying, as the thymol pungency in oregano is brought out and the camphor bitterness in marjoram sharpens and its sweetness deepens.

Both herbs retain their warming power in the dry state, which means they make good herb teas. Julie finds oregano tea light and refreshing in removing the dull heaviness of a headache. Tinctures and the essential oils of both plants are stronger still, and the concentrated oils should only ever be used externally, as a rub for muscle pains or rheumatism, and as an antiseptic or antifungal.

Some of the previous uses of these herbs are little found today. In England's cities in the sixteenth and seventeenth centuries sweet marjoram was everywhere, carried in nosegays, strewn among the rushes on floors, put in sweet bags and added to water. The sweet bags were stored with the family linen or put under the pillow to improve sleep, and oil from dried plants used to polish furniture.

Marjoram powder drawn up into the nostrils was a snuff of choice; in *All's Well That Ends Well* Shakespeare has Lafeu refer to sweet marjoram as a 'nose herb'. Culpeper in 1653 noted that it 'provoketh sneezing, and thereby purgeth the Brain'; when chewed it 'draweth forth much Flegm'.

Here is one herbal area that remains current. Both herbs are used as expectorants for bronchial infections and catarrh, along with chest coughs – they cut and help eliminate phlegm and thereby ease the breathing. Both are also digestive tonics (think oregano on pizza), while also settling flatulence and colic.

The tea can be used to gently ease painful gastroenteritis

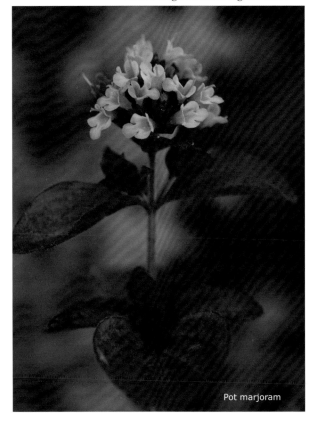

Pot marjoram

and candida. They also make mouthwashes and gargles for sore throats (swill and swallow a cooled tea made of the dried leaves, with honey to taste). This tea, served hot, is also valuable at the onset of a 'flu, or used externally in the bath and as an antiseptic skin massage for eczema or fungal nails. The cold tea, or essential oil, can be rubbed on the temples when a migraine threatens or for a head cold. Raising the core body temperature by drinking hot oregano tea helps restore an irregular menstrual flow suppressed by cold.

Comparing the herbs, American herbalist Peter Holmes, an authority on herbal energetics, finds oregano is the stronger uterine stimulant (hence to be

avoided in quantity during pregnancy), is a more effective respiratory relaxant and expectorant, incites sweating more quickly and has deeper antiseptic and analgesic properties. This bears out the truism that the more southerly and hotter the summer the stronger will be the volatile oils in aromatic herbs.

Oregano leaves

They [oregano tops] are best taken in infusion: they strengthen the stomach, and are good against habitual colics: ... in head-achs, and in all nervous complaints: and they open obstructions, and are good in the jaundice, and to promote the menses.
– Hill (1812)

It [marjoram] is good against the head ach, and dizziness, and all the inferior order of nervous complaints.
– Hill (1812)

Oregano tincture
Steep 3 tablespoons of **dried oregano leaves** in 100ml (3½ fl oz) **white wine** for a month to make a tincture. It is strong, so dosage is a teaspoon three times a day.

Marjoram or oregano tea
Bruise a teaspoonful of **marjoram** or **oregano leaves** and pour on boiling water. Cover and steep for up to five minutes.

Marjoram conserve
This is a recipe by John Nott, cook to the Duke of Bolton, published in London, 1723.
Take the tops and tenderest part of Sweet Marjoram, bruise it well in a wooden Mortar or Bowl; take double the Weight of fine Sugar, boil it with [some] Marjoram-water 'till as thick as Syrup, then put in your beaten Marjoram.
It would work equally well for oregano, the idea being to use bruised herb tops and boil them down in a sugar solution to a syrup. Presumably the 'marjoram water' is optional and ordinary water is sufficient for boiling. The resulting syrup will keep for some months.

Oregano tincture
• infections
• foggy-headedness
• headache
• cough
• bronchitis
• digestion

Marjoram or oregano tea
• digestion
• foggy-headedness
• headache
• cough
• bronchitis
• mouthwash

Marjoram conserve
• sore throat
• cough

Parsley

Petroselinum crispum, P. sativum

Parsley deserves to be more than a garnish, and we should use it often in our kitchens and as medicine. It is one of the most nutritious culinary herbs and a gentle, health-building tonic for the whole body. Parsley is beneficial for the urinary system and the digestion, but also helps relieve gout, rheumatism and arthritis.

Apiaceae (Umbelliferae) Carrot family

Description: Biennial, upright, to 75cm (30in), with pleasant 'green' smell, yellow flowers and dark green, divided leaves.

Distribution: Native to eastern Mediterranean, now cultivated worldwide in temperate areas.

Related species: See text (this page) for cultivars and box opposite for Apiaceae relatives; fool's parsley (*Aethusa cynapium*) is similar in appearance but has a noxious smell and is poisonous.

Parts used: Whole plant, roots, stems, leaves, seed.

The name *Petroselinum* translates as 'rock celery' in Latin, and was eventually abbreviated in English to 'parsley'.

This was a heroic plant for the ancient Greeks, being worn in the victor's crown in the Isthmian games, and also used in funeral wreaths. The Greek term 'to be in need of parsley' meant to be at the point of death.

This dual ritual role gave rise later to superstitions regarding the plant's sowing and transplanting: in the Middle Ages, reports Palaiseul, if you said your enemy's name when plucking a root of parsley he would suffer sudden death. Some people still hesitate to transplant parsley as it might bring them bad luck.

But it was always too useful a plant to succumb to such beliefs. It was valued in classical Greece and Rome as aiding the digestion, as a diuretic and to promote menstruation, more than its uses in cooking.

Today parsley is probably the most popular herb in Europe and North America. It is used almost as a vegetable in Middle Eastern cuisine, but is replaced in India and further east by coriander.

Parsley is conventionally added to salads at home and in restaurants to sweeten the breath, leaving a fresh, chlorophyll taste. It will even remove the odour of garlic, although the French have a sauce, *persillade*, that features both together. The British, since at least Henry VIII's time, have preferred a white sauce with parsley.

The three main cultivars grown for the table are curly-leaved parsley (var. *crispum*), flat-leaved or Italian (var. *neapolitanum*) and turnip-rooted or Hamburg parsley (var. *tuberosum*).

The curly form is generally favoured in the Anglo-Saxon world, often as a raw garnish rather than cooked, while the richer flavour of the flat-leaved form appeals to Mediterranean and Middle Eastern palates for cooking – as in tabbouleh. The large-rooted Hamburg variety is not sold in many garden centres but can be found in specialist seed catalogues.

Given its culinary – and medicinal – value when used fresh, we are lucky that parsley is so easy to grow in most gardens, or in window boxes, has a long season and survives mild winters (the flat-leaved form is the hardiest). Cheap, tasty and useful – a wonderful combination!

Use parsley for...

All parts of the plant are rich in vital minerals (including boron and fluoride), and parsley contains more iron than any leafy green vegetable. It is especially high in vitamins A and C, and contains the essential oils apiole and myristicin, as well as flavonoids.

It is a pharmacopoeia in itself, and eating a few leaves of fresh parsley a day is far more beneficial than an apple! So in a restaurant, make sure you eat the parsley garnish, even if you don't like the food.

The chief vertue of Perslie is in the roote, the next is in the seede, the leaves are of the least force, yet of moost use in the kitchin. ... verie convenient for the stomacke, and stirreth up appetite and maketh the breath sweete.
– Coghan (1584)

It has been found to be almost infallible as a general remedy for bladder infections.
– Wood (2008)

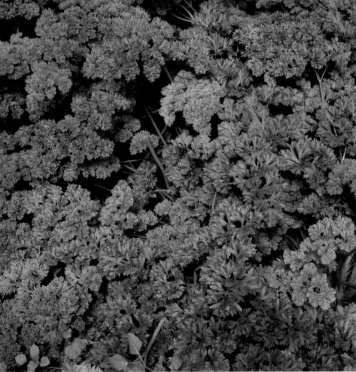

The useful umbellifers
The Apiaceae are an important botanical family for kitchen medicine. We cover some in these pages and wish we could have written on them all:
- alexanders
- angelica
- caraway
- carrot
- celery
- chervil
- coriander
- cumin
- dill
- fennel
- lovage
- parsley
- parsnip
- sweet cicely

The illustration could be an aerial shot of the rain forest but is actually a close-up of parsley tops

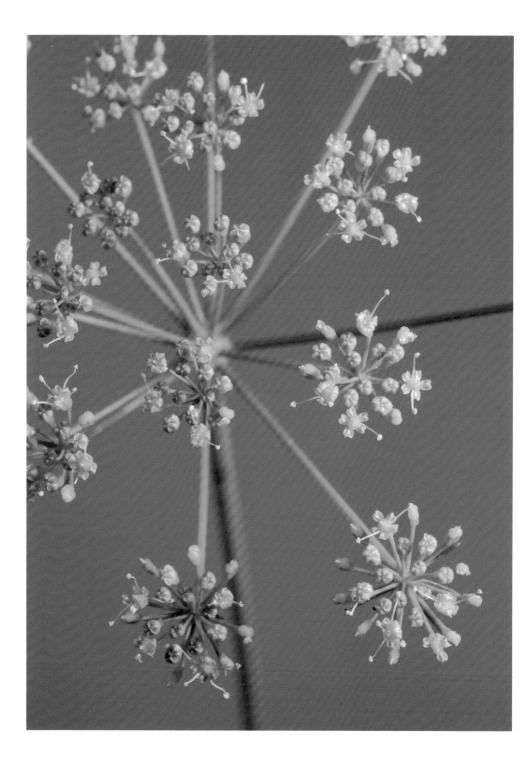

As a biennial, the seeds (fruits) are harvested at the end of the second year; the leaves can be taken at any time. Juice the whole plant as another way to ingest it (it's too strong to take in other than small doses).

The mineral wealth of parsley makes it a bone-strengthener and good osteoporosis supplement. It is also a proven diuretic that can be safely taken to treat gout, rheumatism and arthritis, its scouring action helping flush waste products out of affected joints. Living up to its old name, it can replace celery in these actions.

The seeds, as with other medicinal members of the Apiaceae, are the parts richest in volatile oils and make the strongest diuretic. They are used, especially in Germany, for kidney and urinary tract complaints and to promote menstruation. Parsley, taken as a tea or tincture, is a specific for bladder infection and cystitis.

In the language of the *British Herbal Pharmacopoeia* (1996), the dried leaves and root of parsley are 'official' as a diuretic and carminative, ie to regularise the the urine and digestion.

According to American herbalist Dr Christopher, parsley is a tonic herb for the adrenal glands, the optic nerves and the whole sympathetic nervous system.

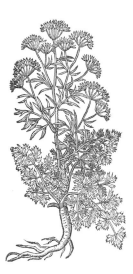

Parsley, from Gerard's *Herball* (1597)

Parsley tea
Chop 1 tablespoon fresh **parsley**, or use 1 teaspoonful dried parsley. Pour a cup of **boiling water** over it, cover and infuse for 5 minutes. Strain and drink hot.

Take often during the day, for menstrual cramps, to aid digestion and stimulate the circulation. This tea can also be used cold as an eyebath.

Parsley root decoction
Boil a tablespoon of fresh **parsley roots** in a saucepan with a large cup or mugful of **water**, for 5 minutes; strain and cool. Drink frequently for kidney or bladder pain, urine retention, oedema or arthritis.

Parsley jelly
Collect about 50 sprigs of **parsley**, place in a saucepan with enough **water** to cover them and add **peel of a lemon**. Simmer slowly for one hour. Strain into a basin. Add **juice of three lemons** and one measure of **sugar** for one measure of the liquid. Heat again until it starts to set.

Store in sealed jars and take in small quantities.

Parsley tea
- cystitis
- weak digestion
- menstrual cramps
- cold, as an eyebath
- circulation

Parsley root
- bladder pain
- cystitis
- urine retention
- oedema
- arthritis

Parsley jelly
- cystitis

Caution: Note that if taken in large quantity parsley seeds, and the essential oil derived from them (apiol), can cause uterine contractions; they should not be taken in pregnancy. Too much parsley can stop lactation.

Pepper *Piper nigrum*

Piperaceae
Pepper family

Description: A rain forest climbing vine, to 4m (13ft), trained by growers through trellises and trees; deep green oval leaves; minute white flowers on hanging catkins; small round fruits, in tight spikes, 20–30 per catkin, the peppercorns, ripening from green to yellow and pinky-red; all stages are used commercially.

Distribution: Native to Malabar, SW India; cultivated in other tropical forests, principally in Vietnam, Indonesia and Brazil.

Related species: Economically significant *Piper* species include two long peppers, the Indian (*P. longum*) and Javanese (*P. retrofractrum*); tailed, cubeb or Java pepper (*P. cubeba*); the betel leaf (*P. betle*), and kava kava root (*P. methysticum*).

Non-related 'peppers': Sichuan pepper or prickly ash (*Zanthoxylum piperitum*); allspice, Jamaica pepper (*Pimenta dioica*); Peruvian pepper tree (*Schinus molle*) and Brazilian pepper tree (*Schinus terebinthifolius*).

Parts used: Fruit, essential oil.

Pepper is 'king of the spices' and one of the oldest traded spices from the East. Seeking a direct route to the source of supply fired the European age of exploration from the late fifteenth century. Nowadays pepper is a condiment found on most kitchen and restaurant tables around the world, and has some useful, if neglected medicinal applications.

When Vasco da Gama sailed around Africa in 1498 and came ashore at Calicut in the south of India, he is reputed to have exclaimed 'for Christ and for spices'. Not quite 'one small step for man', but still a good sound-bite. It was an accurate statement of Portuguese intent: he was after souls and a supply of pepper.

The old overland spice routes from China and India, and the Indian Ocean journey from India via Egypt, with manhandling of products across Suez, were dominated by middlemen, especially the entrepôt monopolies of Alexandria, Constantinople and Venice. These strangleholds could now be broken.

Pepper still accounts for at least a quarter of world trade in spices in any given year, even if Vietnam often out-exports India. Related *Piper* species cubeb pepper and long pepper are no longer significant products, but black pepper (*P. nigrum*) has remained

a staple of world trade for most of recorded history. Here is Pliny, almost two thousand years ago, bemoaning the cost of Indian trade to Rome: '... there is no year in which India does not drain the Roman Empire of fifty million sesterces'. Pepper was a luxury seasoning: the historian of Rome, Edward Gibbon, described it as 'a favourite ingredient of the most expensive Roman cookery'.

In medieval Europe, when other spice delights, like galangal (*Alpinia galanga*) or saffron (*Crocus sativus*) emerged, pepper would fall in esteem, but it was too useful a pungency, too irresistible to the taste buds, to be abandoned. It was easily stored and kept its flavour until crushed; and it came in several forms, offering subtle variations in aroma and taste, which have altered little.

Green peppercorns are picked first, unripe, then pickled in brine; **black** peppercorns are picked unripe, then dried; **red** are

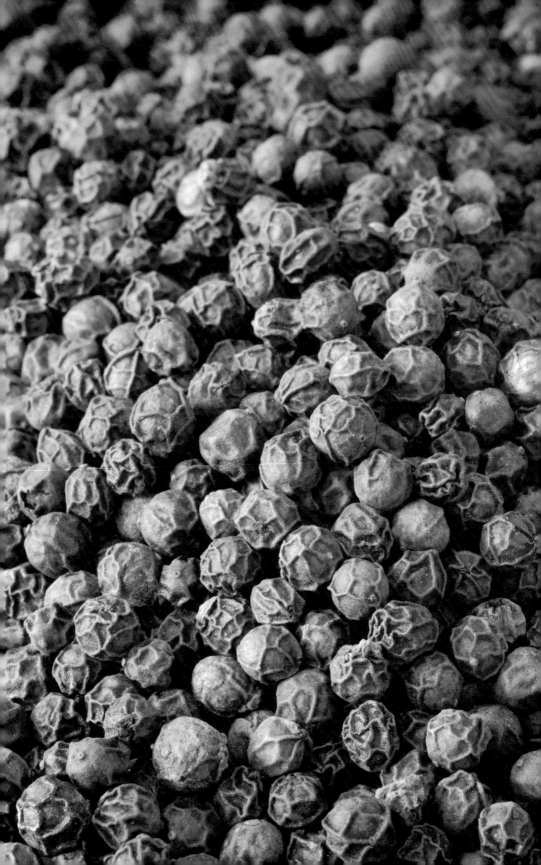

It is remarkable that the use of pepper has come so much in favour ... to think that its only pleasing quality is pungency and that we go all the way to India to get this!
– Pliny (1st century AD)

[pepper is] ... of universal use to correct and temper the cooler Herbs, and such as abound in moisture; it is a never to be omitted ingredient of our Sallets.
– Evelyn (1699)

Cautions
Too much pepper taken at once may overheat the system, with reddening of healthy skin, sweating and possible faintness. As we all know, pepper can be an irritant to the eyes and nose. The answer in all cases, as John Chamberlayne wrote in 1689, is that pepper 'loses most of its hurtful qualities by a moderate use thereof'.

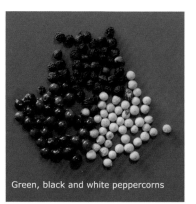

Green, black and white peppercorns

picked ripe, then dried; **white** are picked ripe, steeped in water for a week ('retted'), the outer layer or pericarp removed, and dried. White pepper is the core of the fruit, the volatile and aromatic oils of the pericarp being shed, but the fierce pepper 'bite' retained.

Green corns are fresh and hot, a foodie favourite of the moment; black pepper has a warming and 'robust oiliness', as one spice historian puts it; the white is hotter, 'mustier' (from its fermentation) and sharper to the taste, and the red mellower and almost fruity by comparison.

Today pepper has made the leap from luxury spice to necessary condiment, found on kitchen and restaurant tables around the world. A linguistic sign of its altered state, now universal and costing little, is that a peppercorn rent, once a property more valuable than money itself, now means mere pennies or cents.

Use pepper for ...

Pepper is a supreme digestive stimulant. Its aroma tickles the appetite and causes salivation in anticipation of pungent taste; the pungency itself warms the tongue; and the gastric juices and enzymes are activated. These are invariable, almost reflex reactions.

Not surprisingly, the leading use of pepper medicinally in Ayurveda, India's science of life, is for digestion. Pepper is taken for low appetite and sluggish digestion, to relieve stomach pain and expel toxins. In India, pepper is an anorexia treatment, stimulating hunger and an interest in food. Pepper greatly increases the absorption of other herbs and foods, another reason to use it.

Pepper induces sweat and raises fevers. In Ayurvedic terms, it 'cooks' pathogens, normalising digestive fire and restoring core body heat. It is also taken for intermittent fevers, eg malaria. Pepper benefits a compromised respiration, and is an expectorant for sore throat, asthma, bronchitis and pneumonia. One Ayurvedic measure to clear a blocked nose is to infuse black pepper with ghee. Like rosemary, cardamom and basil, pepper is a 'head' herb.

Pepper stimulates the circulation, notably the micro-capillaries, and crushed black corns, which contain oil, or the essential oil, are rubbed on the skin for muscle pain and, when brave, an aching tooth.

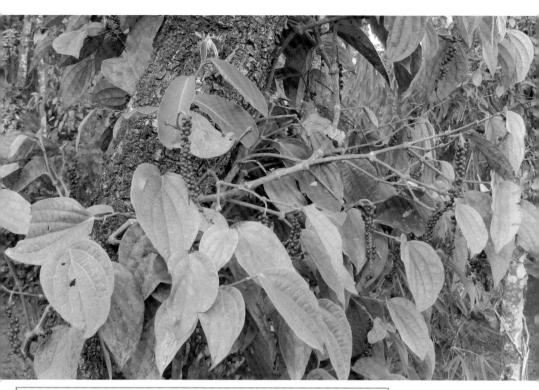

A vegetarian mulligatawny soup

Mulligatawny is an Anglo-Indian soup, the name a corruption of the Tamil for 'pepper-water'. Often made with chicken or mutton, this modified vegetarian version blends a spice paste and vegetables.

Put spice ingredients into a large pot: 5cm (2in) grated **fresh ginger**, 1 small sliced **onion**, 4 cloves crushed **garlic**, 2 small **chillies**, 2 teaspoons each of **curry powder**, **turmeric**, **cumin** and **black pepper**. Cook in 1 cup of **coconut milk** and a little **oil** on low heat for 15 minutes.

Make a **vegetable stock**: 2 sticks celery, 1 medium carrot, 2 medium potatoes and 1 medium onion in boiling water with cilantro and lemon juice to taste. On medium heat this will take about 20 minutes.

Combine spices and stock in one pot, bring to boil and simmer for up to 30 minutes. Serves two or three people. Vary ingredients to taste.

Quatre épices

A classic French 'four spice' recipe to accompany savoury dishes: grind 3 parts **black peppercorns** and 2 parts **cloves** in a coffee mill or spice grinder; empty into a bowl and add 2 parts grated **nutmeg** and 1 part ground **ginger**. Mix thoroughly and funnel into a jar.

Some people add allspice as a fifth element (for a sweeter edge), and others vary the proportions. Experiment and find your own best mix.

Mulligatawny soup
• digestion
• circulation
• coughs
• colds & chills

Quatre épices
• digestion
• circulation
• coughs
• colds & chills

We are apt to neglect things as medicines, that we take with food; but there is hardly a more powerful simple of its kind than pepper, when given singly, and on an empty stomach.
– Hill (1812)

Pineapple *Ananas comosus, A. sativa*

**Bromeliaceae
Bromeliad family**

Description: Tropical perennial growing to 1m (3ft), with sword-like leaves and a single large yellow-fleshed fruit made up of 200–300 fused flowers, each 'spine' being a single flower.

Distribution: Native to South America, now grown commercially in the tropics, principally Hawaii and Malaysia.

Parts used: Flesh, juice, skin.

... [the inhabitants did] *bring us down victual,* [foodstuffs] *which they did in great plenty, as venison, pork, hens, chickens, fowl, fish, with divers sorts of excellent fruits and roots, and great abundance of pinas* [pineapples], *the princess of fruits that grow under the sun, especially those of* Guiana.
– Raleigh (1595)

Pineapple, like pawpaw, is one of the best anti-inflammatory agents in nature. It is both demulcent (soothing inflammations inside the body) and emollient (soothing them outside).
– Elliot & De Paoli (1991)

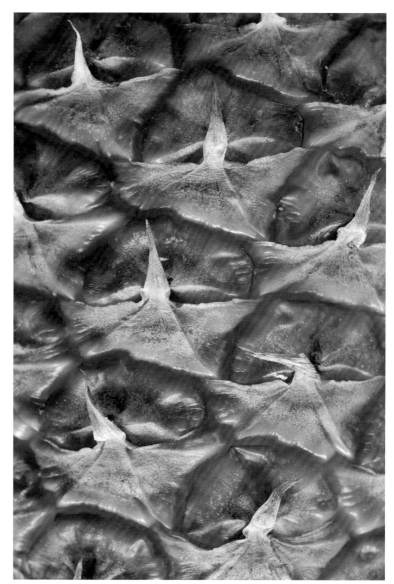

Pineapple ripens from acid to sweet, and from harsh to luscious, carrying the heat of the tropics, but is still not to everyone's taste. Fresh pineapple offers excellent natural medicine, and those who pass it by deprive themselves of a nutritious digestive tonic and safe anti-inflammatory, with fashionable applications as a skin cream and slimming aid.

Pineapple, a wonder fruit when first introduced to Europe from the Americas, is still an intriguing mixture of hard edge outside and soft flesh within. It is sweet but also acidic; it has plentiful minerals, vitamins A and C, and nutritious fibre, but also contains a powerful enzyme that works as a digestive tonic (which explains fresh pineapple juice at breakfast).

This enzyme, bromelain, is a prodigious protein-eater, so pineapple plantation and cannery workers, who handle the plants all day, must wear gloves to protect their hands. Pineapple juice is used as a meat tenderiser. Heat, however, denatures bromelain, so canned pineapple, which has been pasteurised, keeps its taste but loses any medicinal effectiveness.

Fresh pineapple juice is a well-proven anti-inflammatory, safe for both internal and external use. When applied to the skin it will reduce swelling: one research study found it relieved boxers' bruises. It is a folk remedy for corn removal (see panel), and applying the juice soothes tendon pain, so pineapple can be of benefit for tendonitis and bursitis.

A rejuvenating skin cream is made from the juice, and ethnobotanist James Duke suggested using it fresh for wrinkles. Pineapple peel and core are liquefied, and the mash is kept on the skin for half an hour before rinsing it off.

Duke advised eating fresh pineapple for arthritis, gout and allied conditions, saying: 'if you need an excuse to indulge yourself with fresh, ripe pineapple, this is it'.

The juice is a pleasant-tasting gargle for sore throats, and it soothes the whole digestive tract. Pineapple's high satiety index compared with most fruits makes it a boon for slimmers, and slimming capsules are made from the stems, which contain the highest concentrations of bromelain.

Among other medicinal attributes pineapple is cooling for fevers and reduces indigestion and most intestinal upsets. It has also been used for treating burns and ulcers. It is a nutritious food for convalescents and people suffering from iron-deficiency anaemia.

The Brazilian Indian name for pineapple, *nana*, meant 'excellent fruit', and medicinally it earns the title.

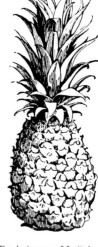

The 'princess of fruits' was Sir Walter Raleigh's description of *pinas* or pineapples, on encountering them in Guiana in 1595

Pineapple
- weak digestion
- indigestion
- bloating after eating
- bruises
- sore throats
- anaemia

A folk remedy for corns
Cut a strip of peel from a pineapple, and attach the fleshy side to the corn by a skin adhesive. Leave overnight. In the morning, soak the foot in hot water and remove any spare skin. Repeat several times until the corn is gone.

Poppy seed *Papaver somniferum*

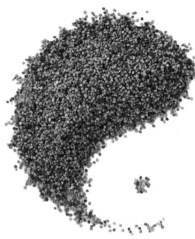

The poppy seeds used in cooking come from one of the oldest medicinal plants known to man, the same plant that produces morphine, codeine and opium. The seeds are prized for their oil content, and for the lovely crunchiness they add to curries, breads, cakes and pastries. They also make a remedy for insomnia.

Papaveraceae
Poppy family

Description: A robust annual growing to about 1m (3ft), with bluish-green leaves. Flower colour can vary from dark red through pink and purple to white.

Distribution: Native to western Asia, cultivated around the world for its seeds (and the oil pressed from them) and as the source of morphine and codeine, as well as for the illegal production of opium and heroin.

Parts used: The seeds are the only part used in cooking.

The tiny black, bluish or white poppy seeds used in cooking around the world are produced by the opium poppy. While the ripe seeds themselves do not contain any narcotic alkaloids, there may be trace amounts on the seeds adhering from the capsule.

The seeds are frequently used in baking, for bagels, bread rolls, cakes and pastries. Poppy seed pastries are often served at Christmas and other festivals. In Europe we normally like the 'blue' black seeds, whereas in India the white seeds are preferred. There they are used in curries and savoury as well as sweet dishes.

Poppy seeds are harvested when the seedheads are ripe, whereas the opiates come from the sap of unripe seed capsules. The seeds are high in oil, which is pressed commercially for use in foods, paints and animal feed.

Even a hundred years ago, opium and its tincture, laudanum, were widely used household remedies and frequently given to children. These products are no longer legal, but morphine remains the best pain relief known to man and is used in hospitals and hospices.

In Ayurveda, poppy seed is considered to be aphrodisiac and tonic, and it is used as a treatment for insomnia. The abundance of the tiny seeds is a symbol of fertility, and their high oil content makes them highly nutritious.

Poppy seed is a home remedy for insomnia, mixed with honey.

Poppy seed electuary
• insomnia

Poppy seed electuary
Grind **poppy seeds** to a powder, then mix into a paste with **honey**.

Take a teaspoonful in the evening to help induce a restful night's sleep.

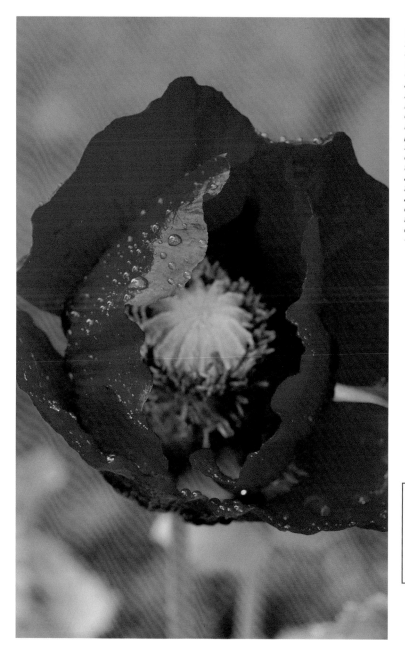

There is no herbal medicine more extensively used, as well as abused, than Opium, and though a valuable remedy, its indiscriminate use is pernicious, as it is capable of doing great harm. Laudanum and paregoric are the forms mostly used in domestic practice, but the 'soothing syrups' and 'carminatives' found in every nursery and household all contain Opium in some form, and work a great deal of mischief.
– Phelps Brown (1907)

Warning: Poppy seeds are banned in some countries. Eating poppy seeds, even the few scattered on top of bread, can sometimes give a false positive on drug tests.

Pumpkin *Cucurbita pepo*

Cucurbitaceae Melon family

Description: Annual vine with prostrate shoots up to 10m (30ft) long, broad lobed green leaves, yellow flowers and large rounded fruit, often orange, with flat, nutritious seeds.

Distribution: North American native, now cultivated worldwide and in gardens.

Related species: Winter squash (*Cucurbita maxima*), squash (*C. moschata*), both also known as pumpkins.

Parts used: Seeds, flesh.

The poor people mix the fleshy part of the fruit with apples, and bake them in pies. The seeds are excellent in medicine; they are cooling and diuretic.
– Hill (1812)

… the drug has steadily grown in favor, and, properly used, is one of our most efficient and harmless tenifuges [expels tapeworms].
– Dispensatory of the United States (1918)

Nowadays, mostly for treating problems of micturition, especially those associated with benign prostate adenomas.
– Bisset & Wichtl (2001)

Pumpkin seeds were once used as a safe and gentle deworming agent. They are high in zinc and essential fatty acids, which with their diuretic and bladder tonic qualities makes them a good preventative treatment for prostate problems. The flesh of pumpkin is cooling and soothing to intestinal inflammation.

Pumpkin's uses extend beyond smiley lanterns at Hallowe'en and Thanksgiving, or Cinderella's coach at midnight. It was a food of the poor, then became a renowned tapeworm treatment and more recently has been used in prostate problems in the mature male.

The Bible tells us that 'the flesh profits nothing' (John 6.63), and it is much the same for pumpkin, although the soup can be taken even when the stomach is upset or feels inflamed. The seeds are the medicinal part, being high in vitamins, omega-3 fatty acids and minerals, notably zinc. The dehusked seeds are used – the familiar olive green, flat seeds that you buy. If you have your own ripe pumpkin, dry the whole seeds. The plastic-like white husks can be peeled off to reveal the seeds. If you have a vegetable garden, there are huskless or naked seeded varieties of pumpkin available that produce seeds that are ready to eat as is.

The action of prostate drugs and herbs – which also include saw palmetto (*Serenoa repens*), pygeum (*Prunus africanum*) and nettle root (*Urtica dioica*) – appears to be to inhibit the prostate gland from converting one form of testosterone to another. This secondary form is the one that stimulates prostate cell growth and contributes to the frequently found benign prostatic hyperplasia (BPH). Zinc in the pumpkin seeds is thought to support this inhibition process.

Zinc has a range of functions in the body in growth and cell division, in insulin activity, in the metabolism of ovaries and testes, in liver function and as a component of many enzymes. High levels of zinc are found in semen, so sexually active men need higher levels in the diet. Pregnant and breastfeeding women also benefit from an increased zinc intake.

Pumpkin seed is also a diuretic, helpful in maintaining normal urinary function, which is challenged by BPH, with its typical symptoms of a need to urinate frequently at night, dribbling and constricting pain in the bladder. This use of pumpkin seeds for prostate, and associated urinary issues, is 'official' in British and German herbal medicine.

The older use of pumpkin seeds to remove tapeworm and other worms has almost disappeared from western practice, but remains part of Chinese herbal medicine. It was in 1820 that a Cuban, Dr Mongenay, discovered by chance that pumpkin (he used the flesh) mixed with honey, diluted in water and taken regularly for three days, with no other food, and followed by a cathartic, like castor oil or senna, would remove a tapeworm.

This home treatment was cheap, safe and had no side effects, and was used with success even by pregnant women, children and the old. It was so predominant for over a hundred years after its first announcement that the US medical establishment fully adopted it.

The protocol could be varied, with the husked seeds sometimes administered with garlic, or milk replacing the water, and fasting before the treatment, or speeding the whole cycle into one day. Pomegranate rind and male fern root might be added. The critical point was that pumpkin effectively 'anaesthetised' the worm, and then the laxative flushed it away, including the tapeworm's gripping head.

How to use pumpkin seeds...
Simply chew a handful of seeds every day, or if you have prostate problems eat a couple of handfuls. If you want a taste change, sprinkle soy sauce or salt on the seeds and roast them briefly in the oven, either alone or with a similar amount of sunflower and sesame seeds (don't roast too long or you destroy the omega-3, although cooking increases zinc absorption).

Pumpkin seeds
- prostate health
- BPH (enlarged prostate)
- water retention
- pregnancy
- breastfeeding

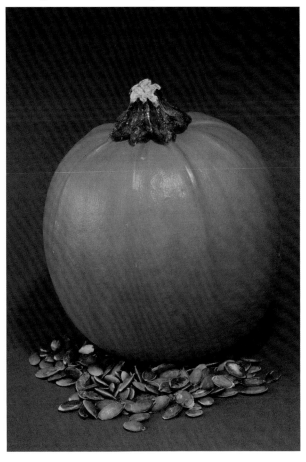

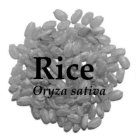
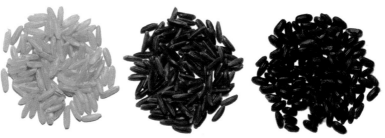

Rice
Oryza sativa

Graminae (Poaceae) Grass family

Description: A domesticated grass, usually grown as an annual crop in warm areas with high rainfall.

Distribution: Cultivated from a wild grass native to Asia, not originally a tropical plant, but now cultivated around the world mainly in the tropics.

Varieties: There are about 8000 varieties of rice grown for food.

Related species: African rice (*O. glaberrima*) has been cultivated in West Africa since pre-Christian times and can be hybridised with Asian rice. Wild rice (*Zizania aquatica*) is not a rice at all but a wild grass native to North America.

In Elizabethan England it [rice] still had a little of the magic of strangeness; steeped in cow's milk with white bread-crumbs, sugar and powdered fennel seed it was given to nursing mothers.
– Davidson (1999)

Rice is one of the most important grain crops in the world, and is the staple food for about half the human beings on Earth. It is one of the easiest grains to digest, making it a good choice for children, the elderly, anyone convalescing and those with food allergies or weak digestion.

The earliest remains of cultivated rice are some 8500 years old, found in the Yangtze valley of China. The Greeks and Romans knew about rice, as an expensive import, mainly used as medicine. It was grown in Egypt by the sixth century AD, and is first documented in England in Henry III's household accounts in 1234.

Rice cooked in clarified butter is said to have been the favourite dish of the Prophet Muhammad.

When rice is harvested, the outer husk has to be removed to make it edible. Often the rice is further polished, making it easier to digest but also reducing the nutritional value. These more polished or white rices are preferred in countries where rice is a staple, but a diet comprised mostly of white rice can lead to beriberi, a disease caused by vitamin B deficiency.

Rice contains no gluten. The so-called 'glutinous' rice is sticky because of its high proportion of the starch amylopectin. Brown rice is sold as a health food in the West and for macrobiotic diets, and it has good levels of B vitamins.

Which rice is best? It all depends on your digestion. If this is strong and can cope with wholegrain rice, it is the most nutritious choice. If, however, your digestion is weak or you have been ill and feel poorly, then go for white rice.

Traditional recipes such as khichri (given opposite) or congee, a rice porridge eaten in China for breakfast, are very easy to digest. Rice pudding can be made with white, black or whole short-grain rice, depending on the state of your digestion, and is nourishing and calming.

Rice has traditionally been used to treat a range of digestive disorders from indigestion to diverticulitis.

Rice types, above from left: short grain, brown basmati, red Camargue and black.

Khichri (kicharee)

Put in a saucepan: 1 cup white **basmati rice** and half a cup **split orange lentils** to 4 cups of water. Add about a quarter of a teaspoonful each of powdered **turmeric, ginger, cumin** and **coriander**. Add a cupful of **chopped fresh vegetables** – whatever is on hand, such as peas, carrots, leeks, spinach or cilantro. Put the lid on, bring to a boil, then simmer gently for 30–40 minutes without stirring. Let it sit for 10 minutes before serving. Add a teaspoon of **ghee** and **salt** and **black pepper** to taste.

This is an ancient Ayurvedic recipe for healing. It is light and easy to digest, yet nutritious, and it helps light the digestive fire. It's a good food to 'fast' on if you are weak, as it will cleanse and give your digestive tract a rest while strengthening the system.

Rice milk

Blend until smooth: 1 cup warm / hot **cooked brown rice** and 4 cups **hot water**. Let it stand for at least 30 minutes. Then, without shaking, pour the rice milk into another container, being careful not to allow sediments at the bottom to pour into the new container. Alternatively, if you are in a hurry, strain it through a cheesecloth.

Rice milk is a good substitute for cow's milk. Try using it in smoothies and milkshakes, or having it on cereal.

Khichri
- convalescence
- weak digestion
- fevers
- detox
- low energy

Rice milk
- convalescence
- weak digestion
- fevers
- dairy substitute
- lactose intolerance

… we tend to overlook the usefulness of rice-water which has long been and still is the classic country remedy for diarrhoea [ie in France]
– Palaiseul (1973)

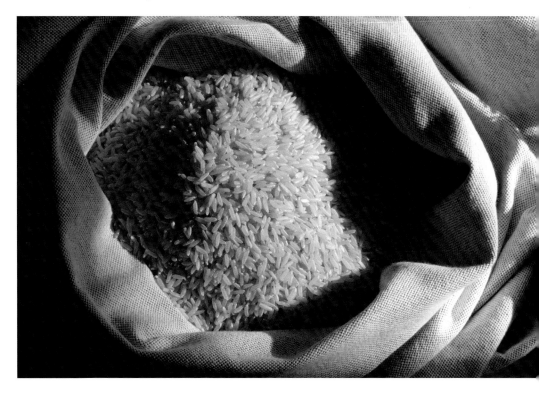

Rosemary *Rosmarinus officinalis*

**Lamiaceae
(Labiatae)
Mint family**

Description: Aromatic, evergreen, perennial, straggling, woody shrub, to 2m (over 6ft), usually less. Leaves simple, spiny, narrow, leathery to about 3.5cm (1½in) long. Flowers pale blue, white to pink, small and lipped.

Distribution: Native to the Mediterranean, spreading to temperate areas worldwide.

Related species: Botanically related to mints and lavender.

Parts used: Fresh or dried leaves and flowers; essential oil.

Rosemary brings into manifestation the full impact on the organism of a Mediterranean plant drenched in cosmic warmth and light, producing powerful, active volatile oils.
– Holmes (1989)

Seethe much Rosemary, and bathe therein to make thee lusty, lively, joyfull, likeing and youngly.
– Langham (1597)

Sovereignly Cephalic, and for the Memory, Sight and Nerves, incomparable.
– Evelyn (1699)

Rosemary is a famed culinary herb with often-overlooked medicinal applications. It brings Mediterranean warmth to the circulation, its pungent aromatic oils tonify the system, and it has multiple restorative properties for the head, stomach, heart and nervous system.

Rosemary is a familiar strongly fragrant herbal presence in gardens, windowboxes and kitchens throughout the temperate world. It was named for its liking of maritime habitats (*ros* was Latin for dew and *maris* for the sea) and, some say, for the way its blue–white flowers have a misty, luminous appearance when seen from a distance. The other half of the scientific name, *officinalis*, indicates the plant's status as a medicinal herb, which has always gone alongside its role in cookery.

It was highly prized by the Greeks and Romans, and the Arab physicians who followed them. The pre-Christian Greeks knew of rosemary's stimulating effect on the blood circulation, and esteemed it for promoting mental concentration. To improve their memories, Greek students wound rosemary strands into the hair when taking examinations, a practice still current in Elizabethan England. You could try the same, using rosemary oil in a burner by your computer as you fill in your tax return: it will calm you as well as keep you mentally agile.

Rosemary became a conventional symbol of remembrance in the sense of fidelity or friendship. Unusually, the plant had a role both at weddings and funerals, as neatly put in a couplet by Robert Herrick (1591–1674): 'Grow for two ends, it matters not at all, / Be't for my bridal or my burial.'

Leaves of rosemary were added to wedding cakes and woven into the bride's chaplet, while at funerals mourners wore sprigs in the procession and dropped these on the coffin. Graves themselves were often planted with rosemary bushes. On Anzac Day, 25 April, in Australia and New Zealand the war dead are still recalled by mourners wearing rosemary.

Other folk uses for rosemary included burning its branches as a fumigant and insecticide. The old French name for the plant – 'incensier' – recalls this. Rosemary was a strewing herb and protective, especially at births.

The herb's old reputation for healing was enhanced by events in medieval times. The later breakthrough was in Spain, in about 1330, with the steam distillation of rosemary oil, which is still used in perfumery and medicinally. A century before that the rejuvenating Queen of Hungary water was developed from rosemary flowers courtesy of a strange 'hermit' (see box).

Use rosemary for...

Squeeze rosemary leaves on the bush or crush dry leaves from your kitchen jar, and you meet a pungent but pleasant, camphor-like aroma. Releasing the locked-in volatile oils is key to medicinal use of the plant, which is why really boiling water is best for making the tea or when preparing a rosemary bath. Another method is to slow-release the oils in a maceration of wine, ale or vinegar, allowing at least two weeks.

The smell is immediately therapeutic. It will 'keep thee youngly', according to *Banckes Herbal* of 1525. A superb antidepressant, rosemary uplifts the mind as it refreshes the body. The Strasbourg herbalist Walther Ryff (1500–48) put it well: 'The spirits of the heart and entire body feel joy from this drink [rosemary wine], which dispels all despondency and worry.'

Whereas old herbals offer multiple rosemary recipes for waters, cordials, conserves, wines or ales, tobaccos and salts, present medicinal use is largely confined to a liquid formulation, whether drunk as a tea or applied

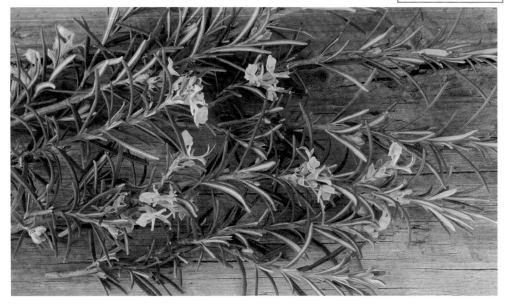

to the body, the essential oil and an infused oil. Losing such diversity is sad, but we can and should still utilise rosemary's qualities.

Rosemary excels as a warming circulatory stimulant, with particular focus on the head, heart and liver. Its hot and drying nature will dispel bodily cold, both when taken internally or applied externally as a massage or compress. It relieves the pain of

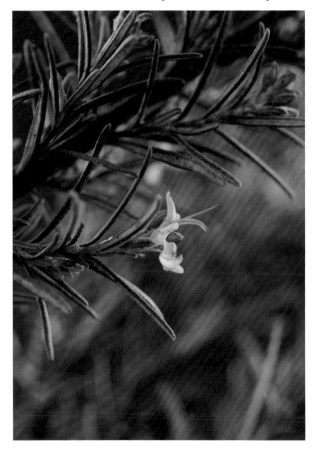

cool conditions, including arthritis and rheumatism, poor circulation and aching muscles. The tea or a rosemary bath promotes sweating and opens sinuses, clearing catarrh and lung colds; it is a good remedy at the onset of influenza.

Rosemary is an important heart herb, unique in its three complementary properties, as one modern herbalist puts it, of being tonic, cleansing and a nervine. Stimulating sluggish circulation warms the whole body, and is one reason why it activates mental processes. Also a relaxant and pain reliever, rosemary is a wonderful headache and migraine remedy.

Modern research explains that rosemary helps maintain the brain chemical acetylcholine. This is a neurotransmitter in the memory area, and low levels of acetylcholine are an indicator for Alzheimer's disease at one extreme, with forgetfulness or lethargy lower down the profile.

Rosemary is a head herb *par excellence*: a Roman treatment for failing eyesight and inflamed eyes; a good breath freshener; rubbed on the scalp, it restores hair and is an excellent shampoo; a refreshing gargle; as Hungary water, a good face wash; mixing sea salt with its leaves is a gentle skin rub.

The stimulating bitters in rosemary tonify the liver and gallbladder, increasing the free flow of bile and digestion of fats (explaining why rosemary is traditionally cooked with lamb). As a moderate diuretic rosemary increases urine flow into the kidneys and raises sweats. Pechey in 1707 used rosemary wine for a 'desperate and slow Diarrhaea'.

Rosemary was also a field wound herb, used as an antiseptic for relieving bruises. The fictional Don Quixote had his wounded ear dressed with a poultice made out of masticated rosemary leaves and salt.

Smudge sticks

Collect some sprigs of **rosemary**, **sage** and **thyme** and use cotton thread to wrap them together into a small stick about a centimetre (½in) thick and 10cm (4in) long. Dry them for a few weeks. To use, hold the end over a candle flame for a few minutes until it becomes red and starts smouldering. The stick can then be carried and waved so that the fragrant smoke wafts around the room.

Rosemary scalp conditioner

Crush 2 tablespoons dried **rosemary** in a mortar and add to a cupful (250g) of extra virgin **coconut oil** in a small saucepan. Heat in a bain-marie (a bath of hot water) for 2 hours. Strain and pour into jars. Massage into the scalp, leaving for 15 minutes or more before shampooing.

Rosemary tea

Add two to six sprigs of **fresh rosemary** tops to a big mug of **boiling water**; cover and allow to infuse for 5–10 minutes. Strain and drink, or use cold as a compress. Good as a general tonic for the heart and liver, for tension headaches and tight shoulders.

Rosemary bath toner

Some formulas suggest boiling about 50g (say 2oz) of **rosemary leaves** or flowers in a litre (1.75 pints) of water, then allowing the mixture to cool and removing the plant before adding the rosemary water to the hot bath. We would simplify this to putting a handful of fresh leaves under the hot tap and leaving them to soak with you. If you prefer, cut rosemary tops with a stalk and bundle them together with a rubber band, making it easier and less messy to remove them from the bath.

Rosemary wine

Take a bottle of **red wine** (or white wine if you prefer) and drink a glassful to make room in the bottle, then add 4 sprigs **rosemary**, an aril of **mace**, a few slices of fresh **ginger** root and a small **cinnamon stick**. Steep for two weeks, then strain through muslin, and rebottle. A wineglassful a day is a tonic after illness and for poor circulation.

Smudge sticks
- freshen the air
- clear unpleasant smells
- warm and clear the atmosphere

Scalp conditioner
- itchy scalp
- dandruff
- tension headaches

Rosemary tea
- warms and clears
- tension headaches
- memory
- concentration

Rosemary bath toner
- warms and clears
- reinvigorates

Rosemary wine
- convalescence
- poor circulation
- debility

Caution:
Rosemary's action as a circulatory stimulant means it is a moderate aphrodisiac and in women stimulates the uterus. Its use in pregnancy should be curtailed, to avoid any risk of abortion. In some women it can bring on heavy periods.

People with high blood pressure should not use rosemary to excess. Do not take rosemary tea before sleep.

Sage *Salvia officinalis*

Sage is a powerful aromatic herb with an impressive healing reputation. Formerly known as 'sage the saviour' and an 'elixir of life', its energetic effects are stimulating and drying, with applications as varied as enhancing the memory, reducing night sweats, allaying sore throats, and support of the nervous and immune systems.

Lamiaceae (Labiatae) Mint family

Description: A small shrub, up to 70cm (27in) high, woody and branched stem, grey–green leaves, flowers violet blue with extending lower lips.

Distribution: Native to the Mediterranean, especially Greece and the Dalmatian coast, now naturalised widely in temperate areas; an important herb in Chinese medicine.

Related species: There are nearly a thousand sage species, including Asian red sage, *dan shen* (*S. miltiorhizza*); Greek sage (*S. fruticosa*); diviner's sage (*S. divinorum*) is a psycho-active species from Mexico, currently sold as a 'legal high'.

Parts used: Leaf, essential oil.

A Mediterranean native, sage was sacred to the Romans. The harvest was blessed by priests, wearing white and going barefoot, who offered up sacrifices of bread and wine. Sage was a herb that protected life, and also one that gave it. Roman couples trying to conceive were kept apart for four days, during which both partners drank copious amounts of sage tea, and then resumed their efforts.

The thirteenth-century doctors of Sicily reflected classic thinking and their own in asking, 'why should a man die in whose garden grows sage?' English writer Thomas Coghan in 1584 held that 'such is the virtue of Sage that if it were possible, it would make a man immortall'.

The plant's medieval reputation had outstripped its name. *Salvia* is from Latin *salvere* for 'to be in good health' and 'to save'. Through permutations like *sawge* and *sauge*, it settled as *sage* in English. Four hundred years ago Sir John Harington neatly linked the saving and wisdom meanings:

In Lattin (Salvia) *takes the name of safety,/*
In English (Sage) *is rather wise than crafty./*
Sith then the name betokens wise and saving,/
We count it nature's friend and worth the having.

'Worth the having' is a good English understatement, for sage was grown enthusiastically wherever it could complete its life cycle. For millennia sage has been prized as an ally in the human journey through life – certainly in European and Chinese cultures – a mental stimulant that was the tonic herb of choice for the elderly and recuperating sick.

Sage linked these two cultures in the seventeenth century, when Chinese entrepreneurs once exchanged with Dutch traders three (and in some versions four) chests of China tea for one of sage. The Chinese had a red sage, *dan shen*, whose root was a significant heart tonic, but there was also a market for grey *salvia* leaf from Europe, while China tea was a new fashion in European cities. In each case the crop exchanged was destined for conspicuous consumption by the rich, and both sets of traders made a killing.

Another interesting 'exchange' happened in the Boston Tea Party in 1773, when the 'Mohawk Indians', really disgruntled American rebels in disguise, tipped more than 300 chests of good but taxed British tea into the harbour. What did the locals have to drink in the next few days? Their own sage tea.

Use sage for...

In his book *The Country Housewife and Lady's Director* (1736) the botanical writer Richard Bradley gave precise instructions for making sage tea. The dried herb was to be infused for half a minute in boiling water, whereupon one should pour it off and 'fling away the leaves'. This gave a tea 'of a fine green Colour, and full of Spirit'; left longer, it would go brownish and lose its flavour.

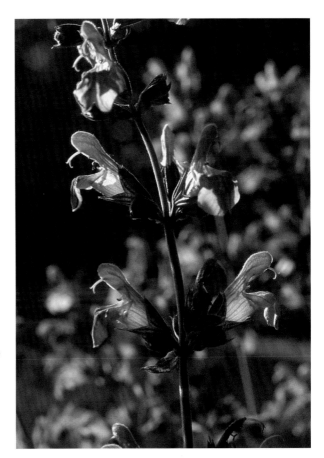

Bradley was right, to a point. The first infusion of sage releases its aromatic oils, which are stimulating ('full of Spirit'), relaxant and antiseptic; these oils boil off as steam after a few minutes. But the later, brownish brew also has a value: it makes available the plant's tannins, with their drying, astringent qualities.

It is the specific combination of stimulation and drying that

underlies the plant's medicinal qualities. Sage's aromatic oils stimulate the pituitary gland, the adrenals, the reproductive hormones and the body's immune system. The tannins help dry excess mucus in the respiratory tract, reduce sweating and can prevent lactation.

This is a herb to be respected and used in moderation, though regular maintenance use of the

... use this [sage wine] *from Michaelmas to the end of March: it will cure any aches or humour in the joints, dry rheums, keep from all diseases to the fourth degree ... sharpens the memory and from the beginning of taking it will keep the body mild, strengthen nature, till the fullness of your day be finished.*
– Mrs Leathe (c. early nineteenth century)

tea has long-term strengthening effects, at menopause, in older age and for the chronically sick. By tradition, the leaves were eaten seasonally: an English country saying was 'eat sage in May, and you'll live for aye', meaning a good span. Sage was a spring tonic, a pick-me-up after winter's dull aches, and May was just before the flowers opened, when the leaves were at an energetic high, fresh, oil-rich and safe.

Sage leaves as a sandwich filling, however, have all but disappeared as a healthy snack – perhaps we are happy enough with sage in cheese: sage derby is flavoured with sage juice and sage lancashire with the leaves. These are strong tastes: as we know from cooking, sage keeps its flavour longer than most herbs, dominating any other taste, and a pinch is enough for slow-cooking meats.

Even taken fresh from the bush sage is an energetic presence. Chewing it brings relief to a sore throat, and rubbing leaves on the teeth whitens them and eases gingivitis in the gums, while leaving the mouth feeling fresh.

Chopping and pulping sage leaves in a mortar produces an effective poultice for wounds, cuts and sores. The dried leaf is an insect deterrent: cut a branch and hang it in your clothes cupboard or burn the leaves as a smudge stick to disinfect a room. These old uses are still effective kitchen medicine.

The tea remains the most popular way to ingest sage, more so than in ale or wine as in times past. Julie finds sage tincture too astringent for most uses, and sticks to the tea, while Austrian herbalist Maria Treben preferred a sage vinegar. Taken before or after meals the tea is digestive, helping to break down fatty foods. It was used as a gargle by the Romans to relieve hoarseness, and, drunk cool with honey and lemon, 'is nearly a specific for sore throat', says Matthew Wood.

Cold sage tea helps the skin retain fluids by reducing night sweats and hot flushes at menopause. As it suppresses lactation, it should be avoided by nursing mothers. It can also improve regularity where there is uneven menstruation through its influence on the pituitary and adrenal glands. Contemporary English herbalist Penelope Ody writes that sage 'could almost be regarded as an early and very gentle form of hormone replacement therapy'.

Sage is also tonic, being good for the heart by stimulating the circulation. In this it resembles rosemary, and is similarly valuable as an antidepressant and for coughs and fevers, not to mention as a hair rinse. Recent research suggests sage as a potential remedy for early stages of dementia. Even if not a herb of immortality, it imparts an abundance of that feel-good factor that improves the quality of life.

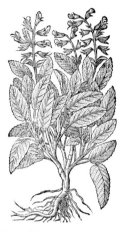

Sage, illustrated in Gerard's *Herball* (1597)

Amongst my herbs, sage holds place of honour; of good scent it is and full virtue for many ills.
– Strabo (AD 840)

Many old people in country districts ascribe their long life and good health to sage tea in spring and autumn, to sage sandwiches for breakfast and supper, or chopped sage added to porridge.
– Ranson (1949)

Sage tea

Use four or five leaves of fresh **sage** or a rounded teaspoon of dried sage per cup of **boiling water**. Make the tea in a teapot or cover the cup to keep the essential oils from escaping. Infuse for about one minute, then strain and drink. The tea can be taken through the day.

Smudge sticks

Collect some sprigs of **sage** (include some rosemary and thyme if you want to) and use cotton thread to wrap them together into a small stick about 1–2cm (½in) thick and 10cm (4in) long. Dry them for a few weeks.

To light, hold the end over a candle flame for a few minutes until it becomes red and starts smouldering. The stick can then be carried and waved so that the fragrant smoke spreads around the room.

Sage vinegar

Put a handful of **fresh sage leaves**, coarsely chopped, in a jar and cover with about a cupful of vinegar. Or use 1 tablespoon dried sage, crushed. Leave to infuse for two to three weeks, then strain and bottle.

For a hair rinse, use 1 tablespoon in a cup of warm water and massage well into the scalp. Leave in the hair for 5 minutes before rinsing out. This rinse darkens hair and leaves it shiny, and helps clear dandruff.

To use as a gargle for sore throats, dilute 1 tablespoon in half a cup of warm water. Honey can be added to taste. Gargle, then swallow.

Sage tooth powder

Mix roughly equal parts **powdered sage leaf** and **bicarbonate of soda**. (You can make your own sage powder by grinding dried sage in a mortar and pestle or an electric grinder, then rubbing it through a fine sieve to remove any large pieces.) Store in a jar to keep dry.

To use, wet your toothbrush, shaking off any excess water, and dip into a little of the powder in your hand (avoid dipping it right into the jar or the moisture can ruin your powder), then brush the teeth as normal. Re-dip the brush as needed.

Rinse your mouth after brushing.

A sage tea is one of the most beneficial to mankind.
– Margaret Roberts (1983)

Sage tea
- hot flushes
- night sweats
- memory
- poor circulation
- sore throat
- warms and clears

Smudge sticks
- freshen the air
- clear odours
- warm and clear
- disinfect

Sage vinegar
- hair rinse
- dandruff
- sore throats

Sage tooth powder
- stained teeth
- gum problems
- bad breath

Caution: *Salvia officinalis* contains thujone, which is toxic in large quantities. It may cause headaches. Do not take medicinal doses while pregnant or breastfeeding.

Salt

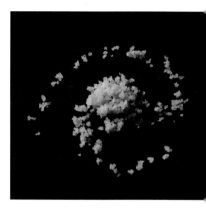

Salt is essential for life, but in recent times has acquired a bad name through the overuse of refined (table) salt. Natural salt contains many valuable minerals and trace elements, and its informed use brings important health benefits and helps avoid lifestyle pitalls.

Description: Salt is normally found in kitchens as a white powder or small crystals. Refined salt is almost entirely sodium choride, NaCl, but natural sea and rock salts also contain other salts such as magnesium chloride.

Source: Salt is either evaporated from sea water or mined as rock salt.

Processing: Most salt for sale in the grocery store will have been refined. It may also have iodine added, and usually contains an anti-caking agent to keep it free-flowing in the shaker.

Other salts: So-called low-salt contains potassium chloride as well as sodium chloride. Epsom salt is magnesium sulphate. Dead Sea salts are quite different from ocean water, being about half magnesium chloride and a third sodium chloride, along with other salts.

Though we have at our command all the spices between Trebizond and Malabar and every aromatic harvested from the Lebanon to Mexico, we cannot ignore our need for salt.
– Elizabeth David (1970)

Salt is a fundamental human need and has always been a vital commodity of trade. It is said that in ancient China the tax on salt brought more money into the imperial coffers than gold. Salt was one of the main items carried in camel caravans to Timbuktu, at the heart of the Sahara.

It is well known that Roman soldiers were paid an allowance for salt. This *salarium argentum* eventually became the English word 'salary'. The Roman term for salt itself, *sal*, came from Salus, the goddess of health (her Greek equivalent, Hygieia, is recalled in our 'hygiene'). Of all the roads leading to Rome, the salt road, the Via Salaria, was one of the busiest, from the salt pans at Ostia to the imperial city and thence east.

'Salt of the earth' is high Biblical praise, and 'worth his salt' goes back to the days when the ancient Greeks bought slaves using salt as a currency.

If you could time-travel to a banquet in medieval England, your status would mean a seat either above or below the salt – the ornamental *saler* or salt cellar. At the same period Venice was growing rich on salt, which its traders exchanged in Constantinople for exotic spices.

Any product vital to life and so valuable a commodity of trade was bound to attract superstition. If you spilled the precious grains, you had to throw a pinch back over your left shoulder. This is the side where evil spirits gathered.

Salt licks are important for animals, and we too need the correct sodium / potassium (or electrolyte) balance in our bodies to maintain health. Sodium and potassium are integral to life as they control the passage of other molecules into and out of all body cells. Salt is necessary for the proper functioning of the adrenal glands, which control metabolic activity.

Potassium is found plentifully in most plant foods, and a good potassium-rich broth can be made by simmering vegetable peelings in water. Bananas are a good source. Sodium occurs naturally in meat and dairy products and vegetables, but salted foods are the main source of our daily sodium needs of about one teaspoon.

A word here about unrefined salt. If the label says 'sea salt', it doesn't necessarily mean it is not refined, so do read the small print. If you can, go for a natural UK sea salt such as Maldon or one of the renowned French and Portuguese salts made the traditional way. In the US choose salts from Hawaii or Maine, and points between.

Once you are used to natural sea or rock salt, you will really notice the harsh metallic taste of ordinary refined table salt, which also contains additives. Salt cravings often disappear when you switch to unrefined salt, perhaps because it was all the minerals in whole salt that you were really missing.

Natural sea salt comprises 95% sodium chloride and 4% potassium chloride. It also contains more than fifty other minerals and trace elements. Interestingly, it has roughly the same balance of minerals as found in human blood. Rock salts vary more in their mineral composition, colour and flavour, but have the advantage of having been laid down before pollution was a factor in the oceans.

Use salt for...

Salt is one of the four basic tastes (with sweet, sour and bitter), and we perceive it in taste receptors in the mouth. Salt brings out the flavour in food by stimulating salivation and helps replenish the body's electrolytes.

Salt works to maintain essential fluids in the body by absorption or 'drawing' across molecular walls – leave salt out in humid weather, and see how it absorbs water until

Modern physiology has demonstrated that an excess of salt interferes with the absorption of nutrients and depletes calcium, whereas appropriate salt usage enhances calcium absorption and nutrient utilization in general.
– Pitchford (1993)

[salt is] ... so great a resister of Putrefaction, and universal use, as to have sometimes merited Divine Epithets.
– Evelyn (1699)

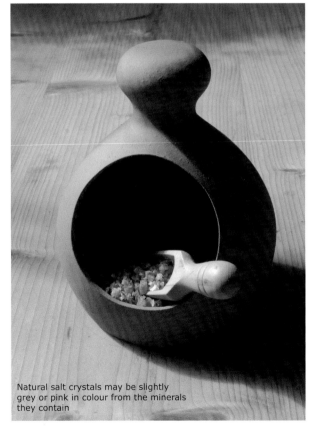

Natural salt crystals may be slightly grey or pink in colour from the minerals they contain

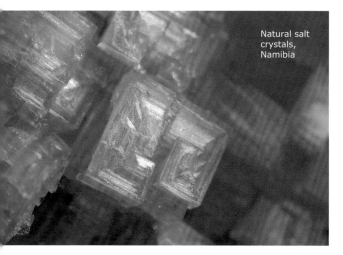

Natural salt crystals, Namibia

In the past fifty years a controversy has raged in the West around salt. Most of the evidence is in, and it shows salt to be a true culprit. However, the salt being tested is not the whole salt used for millennia by traditional peoples but the highly refined chemical variety that is 99.5% or more sodium chloride, with additions of anti-caking chemicals, potassium iodide, and sugar (dextrose) to stabilise the iodine.
– Pitchford (1993)

(opposite) Sea salt being dried, Swakopmund, Namibia, December. The man ran up the salt mound while we took the photo, but we don't know why. Perhaps it was just exuberance, Shakespeare's 'salt of youth'?

the crystals dissolve in their own little puddle.

Salt has always been a vital food preservative, although less significant these days. Its capacity to draw out their cell moisture inhibits micro-organisms from reproducing and hence causing decay in food. By a similar mechanism salt also stops the activity of enzymes that lead to decomposition in food.

It is important to try and maintain the right balance in salt intake, even when many junk foods tempt us with abnormally high salt levels. Manufacturers have reduced amounts, but each of us needs to keep our salt antennae tuned. In some people, salt in the diet is related to high blood pressure, so if you have hypertension try reducing salt intake and see if it helps.

If Julie has a patient suffering with oedema and fluid retention, one of the first things she checks is the person's salt intake. If the level is high, then a simple cut in their salt is often enough to rectify the problem, although of course there can be many other causes.

We recommend using salt crystals in the bath to ease minor aches and pains. Bath salts often combine Epsom salts (magnesium sulphate) with regular salt. Use a good cupful of salt in the bath for the best results, but don't take a salt bath every night as it can be too depleting. Matthew did that once before a marathon race and felt almost too tired to start.

Salt dissolved in water is a traditional solution for washing cuts, abrasions and minor wounds and will help in their healing. A salt solution can also be used as an eye wash, mouthwash and gargle.

Mineral-rich natural sea and rock salts can help relieve muscle cramps, and also help restore electrolytes as part of an oral rehydration solution (recipe, p167).

If you don't believe all of this, you might 'take it with a grain of salt'. This old phrase conveys the idea that you will allow a grain of truth in a statement, as a little salt will help you swallow something. Oddly enough, you need a 'spoonful of sugar to make the medicine go down', which says something about relative values!

Salt gargle

Mix a couple of teaspoons of **salt** in half a mug of **warm water** and stir until dissolved. Use as a gargle for sore throats, or as a wash for minor wounds. It also makes an excellent gum wash.

Rejuvenating hand and body scrub

Put fine **salt** in a jar until nearly at the top, and slowly add extra virgin **olive oil**, stirring until the salt is all covered. You will need roughly equal volumes of salt and oil. This mixture can be scented with 1 teaspoonful **vanilla** extract or a few drops of your favourite essential oils. To use, scoop out a small amount and rub onto dry skin, then rinse with water. This is especially good for the hands after gardening, and to soften and smooth elbows, knees and feet.

Eyebath

Dissolve half a teaspoonful **sea salt** in half a cup of **boiled water**. Allow to cool, then use to bathe the eyes, using an eye cup or a small glass to hold the fluid.

Salt gargle
- sore throats
- wash for cuts
- wash for gums

Rejuvenating hand & body scrub
- after-gardening rub
- rough knees, elbows

Eyebath
- gritty eyes
- tired eyes

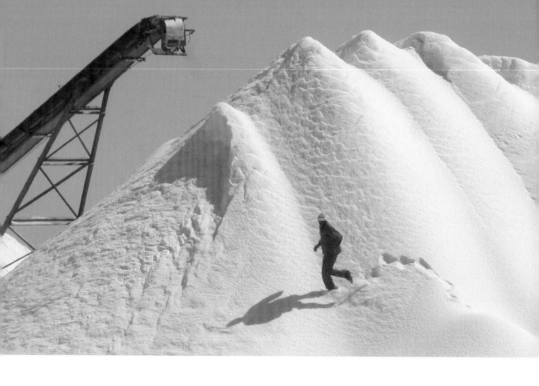

Star anise *Illicium verum*

Chinese anise, Badyan

Star anise has no botanical or even visual connection to anise, but is similar in having high quantities of anethole, which gives it an 'aniseedy' taste, and works equally well for digestive and bronchial problems. Star anise often becomes newsworthy as a natural source of the antiviral Tamiflu.

Schisandraceae
Schisandra family

Description: An evergreen tree growing to 18m (60ft), with small cream flowers followed by woody, eight-pointed fruits with one seed in each section. Hardy to −5°C (23°F).

Distribution: Native to woodland in China and Vietnam.

Related species: There are about 40 species in the genus. Sometimes star anise is adulterated with Japanese star anise (*Illicium anisatum*), which has smaller scentless fruits containing toxic substances.

[Japanese star anise] *is called the 'mad herb' in China, but in Japan it is revered and used at funerals.*
– Stuart (1979)

The first thing to say about star anise is that is completely different from aniseed (see p8 above) in all ways but one, and that similarity happens to be significant. Star anise has eight-winged fruit pods with a round, bronze seed in each segment of the star, while anise has small, cumin-like fruits.

But the interesting thing is that while there is no botanical or visual connection between the two spices, they do both contain high quantities of the compound anethole, the substance that lends them an 'aniseedy' taste and smell, and gives rise to similar commercial and herbal uses.

Commercially, star anise is imported to the West as a cheaper substitute for anise in liqueurs, including Pernod, anisette and pastis, and as a flavourant for coffee and confectionery items, cough syrups and tobacco.

We use it ourselves to give a warm, tingly edge to fruit juices and in Indian-style tea (chai). As it is indigestible in the dried form, be sure to remove it before eating or drinking things you make with it, or keep it in a muslin bag so that you can easily withdraw it.

In Chinese cuisine 'five spice powder', a blend of star anise, cinnamon, cloves, fennel and pepper (ginger, galangal and cardamom are sometimes substituted), is widely used in meat, fish and sweet dishes.

You can experiment with your own combinations of spices, and any mix of these strong tastes will be a lively addition to stews, curries and baked fruit.

Star anise is stronger in taste and aroma than anise, and should be used sparingly in your food or home-made medicines.

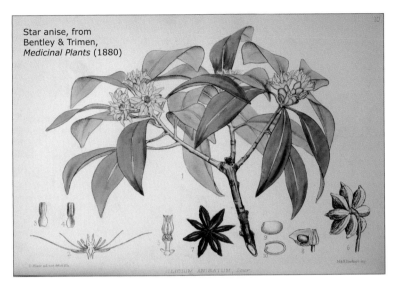

Star anise, from
Bentley & Trimen,
Medicinal Plants (1880)

Star anise and Tamiflu
Star anise is periodically in the news because it has the most concentrated natural source of shikimic acid, which is made into the antiviral drug Oseltamivir, sold under the trade name Tamiflu. In the bird 'flu outbreak in 2005 and again in the swine 'flu pandemic in 2009, provision of stocks of Tamiflu became a charged international political issue. Prices of star anise rose steeply, especially as supplies are limited because the trees grow slowly and the manufacturing process is long and complex, while worldwide demand for the drug soared. Roche, the pharmaceutical multinational that monopolises the industry, has sought alternative sources of supply by turning to the bacteria *E. coli* as a culture in which shikimic acid can be developed.

Use star anise for...

In Traditional Chinese Medicine, star anise is *Ba jiao hui xian* (eight-pointed star or fennel), used dried, either as the whole fruit capsule or ground to a powder. In TCM terms it treats rheumatism, stomach pain and hernias, is a breath cleanser and is given to children for colic.

In western herbalism, uses are similar, and align with those of anise, in digestive and bronchial problems, with emphasis on calming intestinal spasm or hiccups, and helping eliminate phlegm. Herbalist Matthew Wood says he often uses star anise as a specific for congestion in the maxillary sinuses, 'and it has always worked surprisingly well'.

In 2003 the Food and Drug Administration (FDA) in the USA issued an advisory against the use of star anise in teas intended for babies with colic, after several dozen cases of neurological damage were reported. This arose from adulteration, and star anise was absolved, but anise is a wiser choice for small children's use.

Star anise tea

Put two or three of the stars in a mug and pour boiling water onto them. Cover and let steep for about 5 minutes. Drink hot. Incidentally, if you wonder why herbal tea recipes always advise you to cover the brew, it is to prevent volatile oils escaping as vapour.

Star anise tea
- indigestion
- sluggish digestion
- sinus congestion
- nasal catarrh
- rheumatism

Sugar Sucrose

Sugar cane
Saccharum officinarum
**Graminae (Poaceae)
Grass family**

Distribution: Native to India, cultivated in tropical areas including South America and the West Indies, USA, India and Pakistan, China, SE Asia, Philippines and northern Australia.

Sugar beet
Beta vulgaris var. altissima
**Amaranthaceae
Amaranth family**

Distribution: Derived from sea beet, native to Europe, and the main source of sugar in temperate regions of the world.

Other sugars
Glucose is used medically in drip solutions and other applications. It gives a very quick energy boost when taken orally.

The sugar maple tree (*Acer saccharum*) is the source of maple syrup.

In Chinese medicine *Saccharum granorum* (*jiao tang*), barley malt sugar or maltose is used for dry coughs and deficiency, to tonify the *qi*.

We all know sugar helps the medicine go down, but sugar as medicine, you ask? Well, yes! Its ability to kill bacteria, which makes it so useful in preserving jams and syrups, also works on wounds to keep them clear of infection. Sugar saves millions of lives each year when used to make oral rehydration solutions, particularly for children in developing countries.

Sugars are produced naturally by many plants, and include glucose, fructose and sucrose. What we know as sugar is sucrose, with sugar cane and sugar beet the main commercial sources.

Sugar gets a bad press because of the numerous health problems that result from a diet high in refined sugar and other carbohydrates. It also has a muddied past, with the sugar trade being closely linked with slavery.

Sugar cane is thought to have been cultivated in India since 800 BC but took its time to arrive in the west. Arab merchants introduced crystallised sugar as *qandi* (which gives us our word candy) and various products of sugar such as syrups and caramel. Crusaders then returned to Western Europe with sugar in the twelfth century, but it remained an exotic and expensive luxury for hundreds of years. Honey was the local sweetener more readily available, but this was scarce and reserved for special occasions.

By the sixteenth century, sugar was already grown in the New World and imported to metropolitan Europe. Some doctors considered it a dangerous mind-altering drug, and it certainly wreaked havoc with people's teeth.

It took the discovery (in 1747) that sugar beet could be bred to yield as much sugar as imported cane to bring sugar prices within more general reach in Europe. Today we enjoy a rich choice. The unrefined brownish types, like Indian jaggery and muscovado, demerara and turbinado varieties, introduced between the seventeenth and nineteenth centuries, contain more minerals and nutrients than refined white sugar and have richer flavours. These are the better varieties to use in cooking and baking.

Refined white sugar – 'pure, white and deadly', as critics say – is actually superior in preserving foods and as an antiseptic for minor wounds. Simply sprinkle some onto cuts and grazes.

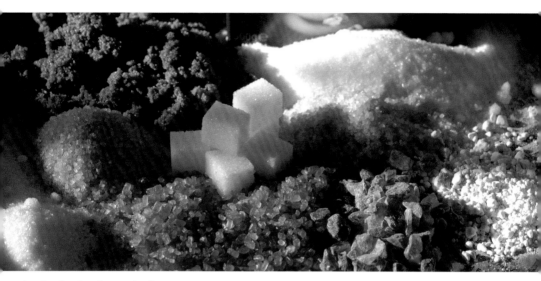

Oral rehydration solution

Mix 1 litre (5 cupfuls) warm **water**, 8 teaspoons **sugar** and ½ to 1 tea-spoon **salt**. Use a raw brown sugar or molasses if available instead of white sugar as these contain higher levels of potassium.

If giving to a child, feed the child slowly after every loose motion, using a teaspoon. If the child vomits it up, try giving it again.

Dose: For a child under two: between a quarter and a half cupful at each feeding. (Note: if the child can be breast-fed, that is ideal, but they may still need some extra fluids.)
For older children: between a half and a whole large cup.
Adults and large children: should drink at least 3 litres a day until they are well.
For severe dehydration: Give sips every 5 minutes until urination is normal. (It's normal to urinate four or five times a day.)

Sugar scrub

Mix ½ cup **white sugar** with ½ cup cold-pressed almond, olive or sesame **oil**. Store in a jar – expensive at a spa, but easy to make in your kitchen. To use, rub into wet or dry skin, working up from your hands to your shoulders, and from your feet up your legs to your torso. Scrub vigorously so that your skin tingles, then rinse off with warm water.

Sugar and soap

Mix a pinch or two of **sugar** with a little soft **soap** (from the wet under-side of a bar of soap is perfect) to make a soft paste. Apply on a splinter, put a plaster over it and leave overnight. In the morning the splinter should come out easily – if it doesn't, reapply some more sugar and soap until it does.

Sugar is temperate, though sometimes inclining to hot, and is good in all sort of Food, except in Tripes; for being put thereon, it makes them stink like the Dung of an Ox newly made.
It nourishes more than Honey, maintains the Body clean, and cleanses it from Flegm, mollifies the Breast, clears the Stomach, is good for the Kidneys, the Bladder, and the Eyes.
– Chamberlayne (1689)

Oral rehydration solution
• dehydration from diarrhoea, vomiting or athletic exertion
• children's diarrhoea
• children's vomiting

Sugar scrub
• cleans skin
• exfoliates
• stimulates circulation
• moisturises

Sugar & soap
• draws splinters

Tea *Camellia sinensis* [older names: *C. thea, Thea sinensis, T. bohea, T. viridis*]

**Theaceae
Tea family**

Description: An evergreen shrub that grows to about 6m (20ft) if left, but normally pruned to 1m (3ft); small, leathery and elliptical leaves and white flowers, with yellow stamens, and large oily seeds.

Distribution: Native to SW China and adjacent areas, now cultivated commercially in India, Kenya, Russia, Indonesia and many other places, even in the British Isles.

Parts used: Young top leaves and buds, handpicked, every few weeks in season.

*The excellent and by all physitians approved China drink, called by the Chineans Tcha, by other Nations Tay, alias Tee.
– Thomas Garway, advertisement for tea at his 'Cophee-House, in Sweeting's Rents by the Royal Exchange', London, in Mercurius Politicus, 23–30 September 1658, the first record of tea for sale in London*

Is it fair to say tea lovers quickly become addicts? Whether you take your tea green and pure or black with lots of milk and sugar you are taking a view on how best to enjoy tea's caffeines and tannins. Medicinally, tea has valuable antioxidant properties as well as use in traditional home remedies.

Tea is second only to water as the world's beverage, and we are with the Rev. Sydney Smith, who said in the early nineteenth century, 'Thank God for tea! What would the world do without tea? How did it exist? I am glad I was not born before tea.'

Most Britons would still agree: the nation currently quaffs over 160 million cups daily, or almost three for every person every day. Some have far more: hands up, you dozen-a-day addicts! Tea accounts for over half the fluid intake of many Britons.

Tea gives humble foods or domestic occasions a warm, ritual blessing. Somebody once expanded this to: 'bread and water can so easily be toast and tea'. The American writer Alice Walker memorably wrote that 'tea to the English is really a picnic indoors'. The stock phrase 'fair to middling', used to describe both personal health and the weather, is a term borrowed from tea-grading. Tea remains the essence of British domesticity.

It is the drink for any occasion, a wake-up call, or with afternoon scones and crumpets, perhaps a companion through the day: in the office or factory, work breaks are still 'tea breaks'.

Tea also met and continues to meet minor domestic medical needs. Hot milky tea with sugar is given everywhere for shock and after fainting; minus sugar or milk it is a remedy for diarrhoea; tea is an aid for slimmers and those with sweaty feet; it helps relieve eye strain and tooth decay. It has more recently established uses as an antioxidant, as we will see.

A cup of tea contains about half the caffeine of coffee, which makes it a mild stimulant with a lift that improves short-term mental alertness. In an Indian legend the Buddha once fell asleep while meditating. This must have been before he was enlightened, because he reacted by tearing off his eyelids, which rooted in the ground and grew into tea plants. The eyelid-shaped leaves had the power to keep you awake.

The caffeine effects extend to the stomach, where it peps up the digestion, as we all know, and the kidneys too, making tea a diuretic as well as an energy booster.

Tea's caffeine dissolves quickly in boiling water, so a quick brew (say up to 45 seconds for a tea bag, two minutes for leaf tea) will be more stimulant in nature. Brewed or stewed tea (over these times) brings out the tannins, which have an astringent and bitter quality. Many people disguise this by adding sugar and milk (builder's tea), which has a comfort factor but 'lacks that antioxidant punch'.

Timing of brew length was already apparent to the earliest English tea lovers. Not long after the first tea shop opened in London, in the 1650s, Sir Kenelm Digby (1669) wrote of a Jesuit who had come from China with some tea recipes (cooked with egg). Sir Kenelm noted that too long a soaking of hot water on the tea 'makes it extract into it self the earthy parts of the herb'. He specified: 'The water is to remain upon it, no longer than whiles you can say the *Miserere* Psalm very leisurely. Thus you have only the spiritual parts of the Tea, which is much more active, penetrating and friendly to nature.' Earthy and spiritual are evocative ways to describe tannins and caffeine respectively.

The three categories of commercial tea – black, green and oolong – are all products of *Camellia sinensis*.

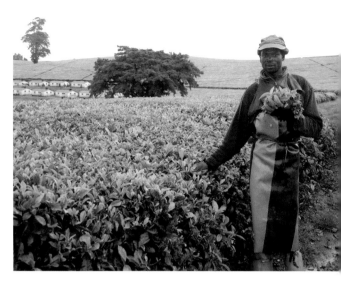

Recent global market breakdown figures show black tea had a 78% share, green 20% and oolong 2%.

Black tea is picked, the leaves wilted, rolled and allowed to ferment in the air and dried. Green tea is unfermented, the picked leaves being steam-dried immediately, preventing oxidation. Oolong or pouchong are larger-leafed teas that are part-fermented.

The degree of oxidation is significant. In green tea, an oxidising enzyme or polyphenol found in black tea has no chance to change the so-called super-nutrient EGCG (in full, epigallocatechin gallate), which means green tea retains plentiful EGCG, or antioxidants. Studies

(above) tea-picking on a rainy day near Nairobi, March; (below) *Camellia sinensis*, from Bentley & Trimen, *Medicinal Plants* (1880)

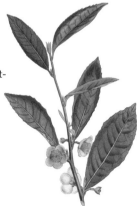

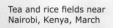
Tea and rice fields near
Nairobi, Kenya, March

have identified three such catechin antioxidants. Black tea, by contrast, is rich in theaflavins and thearubigens, which contribute to its colour and flavour.

Green tea is in fashion, along with estate and fruit teas, and the costly white tea. This is a recent reversal, influenced by research findings into tea's health-promoting qualities. Back in the 1930s, Mrs Grieve allowed that moderate amounts were 'harmless', but excessive quantities of tea produced 'nervous and dyspeptic symptoms, the green variety being decidedly the more injurious'.

Use tea for...
Tea began life being branded as a healing drink. Two examples: British brand Typhoo is from the Chinese word *dai fu*, for doctor; and PG Tips originally stood for 'pre-gest-tee', meaning to be drunk before food was digested.

The astringency in tea readily settles upset stomachs and diarrhoea, the antioxidants attacking infection and improving intestinal tone. This is both a western and a traditional Chinese remedy. For best results use black tea (more tannins), without sugar or milk. A Chinese treatment for gastroenteritis is a mixture of used green tea leaves and dried ginger.

Tea also attacks fat: traditional Mongolian fare is large amounts of meat together with strong green tea. It appears that the tea

burns fat on the stomach and more generally, possibly by the EGCG speeding up the rate of fat absorption. This can be for you as well as Mongolians!

In British folk medicine tea makes a good soother of inflamed or puffy eyes, and comes in a perfect size and shape – the teabag. Simply place a used bag on the affected eye, or if you prefer soak a ball of cotton wool in cold green tea and put this over the eye.

Similarly, tea bags or soaked tea compresses help relieve the pain of sore or inflamed joints, especially ankles, and will soothe an insect bite or other skin irritation. A well-tried application is for sweaty or smelly feet: boil a large pot of tea, let your tea brew and build up tannin levels, then once cool, pour it into a bowl and soak the feet there for half an hour.

Another application of tea in kitchen medicine is to fight tooth decay, the tea's natural fluoride content having this effect in addition to fluoride in the water supply. Naturally, though, adding extra sugar will do more harm than good to vulnerable teeth.

Green and oolong teas, taken in a number of small cups a day, have developed a recent reputation, based on animal research, for controlling cholesterol levels, lowering blood pressure and reducing heart disease. Black tea's theaflavins and thearubigens are

It is true that tea is more used for pleasure than as a medicine, but green tea is diuretic and carries an agreeable roughness with it into the stomach, which gently astringes the fibres of that organ, and gives such a tone as is necessary for a good digestion ... in general, there is very few plants made use of, either as food or medicine, that are better, when used with moderation, or pleasanter than tea. – Meyrick (1789)

I view the tea drinking as a destroyer of health, an enfeebler of the frame, an engenderer of effeminacy and laziness, a debaucher of youth and a maker of misery for old age. – Cobbett (1830)

Grown almost exclusively for use as a beverage, tea is perhaps the world's most undervalued medicinal plant. – Chevallier (2007)

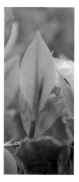

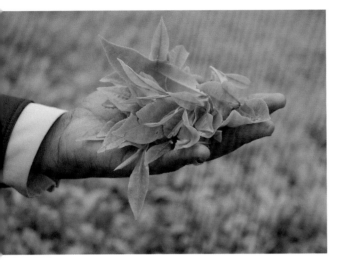

for tea's anti-cancer and anti-tumour activity? 'Encouraging in animal studies, but not proven in human trials' is the present position as research continues. You can't yet say that drinking tea protects you from cancer, but the question is being taken seriously.

Is there a downside in this 'teappraisal'? One area of concern is that tannins, if ingested in large quantity, interfere with iron absorption in the gut, preventing it being fully assimilated. Taking milk or lemon with your tea reduces this tendency. An earlier criticism that excess tea can reduce levels of vitamin B1 (thiamin) seems to be less heard nowadays. But admonitions not to take too much tea during pregnancy or when suffering from peptic ulcers or insomnia should be heeded.

How much caffeine?
A comparison of caffeine in the main non-alcoholic drinks in the typical western diet gave these results in 1996. For a cup of 150ml (1/4pt) or a 125g (4oz) bar of chocolate, with all caffeine figures in mg: ground coffee 100, instant coffee 75; dark chocolate 80, milk chocolate 50; tea 50; colas 40; cocoa 4; decaffeinated tea and coffee 3; rooibos tea 0.

Eye refresher
• tired eyes
• puffy eyes
• sore eyes

Masala chai
• refreshing
• digestion

being researched for reducing stroke and heart attacks.

These are considerable advances on the accepted wisdom of Mrs Grieve's day. And what of claims

Eye refresher
Put used **tea bags** in the refrigerator. For tired eyes, recline with your head and neck resting comfortably and put a cold tea bag over each eye. Leave for a few minutes.

Masala chai
This is traditional Indian spiced tea. It has infinite possible variations, so try the basic recipe and then experiment to see what you like.

In a saucepan, place 2½ cups **water** and 2½ cups **milk** (or almond, soy or rice milk), 3 teaspoons **green tea**, 1 teaspoon **Darjeeling or black tea**, 6 **cardamom pods**, a small piece of **cinnamon** quill, 2 **cloves**, ½ teaspoon **ginger** powder or a couple of slices of fresh ginger, ¼ teaspoon **black pepper** and ¼ teaspoon **nutmeg powder**.

Heat to boiling point, then stew gently for about 20 minutes. Strain and serve hot, adding **sugar** to taste. In India this tea is made cloyingly sweet, being brewed along with the sugar, but adding it at the end gives extra flexibility in the sweetening.

Home Remedies

Thyme
Thymus vulgaris, **Common or garden thyme**

Thyme's original Greek name meant both 'strength' and 'cleansing'. As a herbal medicine it embodies both qualities, especially in treating the respiratory and digestive systems, accompanied by a sweetness and uplifting aroma that are themselves healing and restorative.

Thyme is a small Mediterranean herb with hidden depths. Its old Greek name, *thumon*, meant 'strength' or 'valour', and it does seem to flourish when crushed. It is still planted on paths, and trampling releases its sweet and healing volatile oils.

It also forms a dense, antiseptic smoke when burned – another meaning of its Greek name was 'fumigation' or 'cleansing'. Thyme accompanied the dead in Egyptian and Etruscan mummification, was an incense in Greece and Rome, and a medieval plague protection.

Thyme remains a powerful medicinal presence in western herbalism. Peter Holmes, a contemporary American herbalist, notes that, in common with marjoram, sage and other aromatics, thyme best releases its potential – its 'warm, dry, bitter and pungent principles' – as a tincture or essential oil. Holmes calls thyme tincture a 'superior qi tonic', with particular benefit to the respiratory and digestive systems.

Thyme's strength relates to thymol, its main essential oil, which is twenty times stronger than phenol (carbolic), the standard medical antiseptic. Thymol was first isolated in Germany in 1725 and has been in pharmaceutical use ever since.

Thymol was used to medicate bandages and made a local anaesthetic for dentists. Chewing fresh or dried thyme leaves at home brings emergency pain relief for toothache or inflamed gums. Holmes calls thyme mouthwash 'a stronger anesthetic for mouth, gums and teeth than Clove'.

Thyme's rich chemistry includes the tannins and phenols that make it bitter medicinally, but it also contains an uplifting sweetness that can be tasted and smelled. In ancient Rome thyme was a mainstream remedy for melancholy. Culpeper (1653) said thyme was 'so harmless you need not fear the use of it'. Nonetheless, take due care when using the essential oil, which is very concentrated, and do not ingest it.

Lamiaceae (Labiatae) Mint family

Description: Quick-growing, aromatic 'carpet' herb, prostrate, or a small, woody shrub, with small leaves and pinkish flowers.

Distribution: Native to the Mediterranean and Middle East; wild and cultivated, a culinary and garden favourite.

Related species: Wild thyme (*T. serpyllum*; *T. polytrichus*); lemon thyme (*T. x citriodorus*), and many other varieties.

Parts used: Flowering tops, dried or fresh; essential oil.

Thyme is almost as essential as salt in the diet.
– Margaret Roberts (1983)

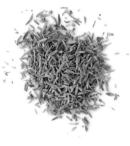

Use thyme for...

Numerous varieties of thyme are grown in gardens but few are as medicinal as common and wild thyme; for most purposes these are interchangeable. Wild or creeping thyme (*T. serpyllum* or *T. polytrichus*) was called 'mother of thyme' well into the nineteenth century. It was known to be the progenitor of common thyme (*T. vulgaris*) and was itself

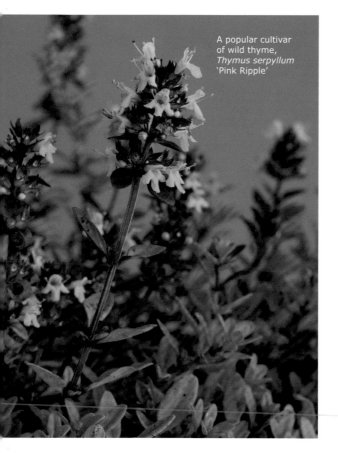

A popular cultivar of wild thyme, *Thymus serpyllum* 'Pink Ripple'

a remedy to treat menstrual disorders. Common thyme is the cook's choice, while lemon thyme (*T.* x *citriodorus*) makes perhaps the tastiest thyme herb tea.

The signature use of thyme is as a respiratory herb, which improves expectoration and relieves coughs and wheezing; it was once a specific for whooping-cough. As an antispasmodic it is beneficial in cases of asthma and bronchitis.

The Greek physician Dioscorides (1st century AD) recommended a thyme tea with honey for a sore throat, and it remains a good remedy. A syrup of thyme made with dried herbs is a wonderfully soothing gargle and antiseptic. Smoke from burning dried thyme was formerly an inhalation for sinusitis, dried leaf was crumbled as a snuff and a thyme bath used to relieve respiratory issues.

Thyme's degree of antiseptic strength was substantiated in nineteenth-century research that showed it to stimulate immunity to dangerous infections including anthrax, typhoid and diphtheria. It was formerly used to combat hookworm and other parasites.

It is equally a digestive herb, which warms and dries a cold stomach and the gastrointestinal tract, soothing colic, indigestion and irritable bowel, and diarrhoea in children. It is heating enough to raise body temperature to fight off fevers. Another area of thyme's action is for nervous relaxation, in conditions of stress, headache, depression and insomnia. It is a uterine herb, for diseases of the uterus and to reduce period pain (it is to be avoided in pregnancy).

Finally, thyme is a readily available immune-supporting herb, with special affinity to the lymphatic system, the thymus gland and spleen. It also clears parasites and toxins.

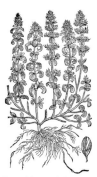
Broad-leaved thyme, from Gerard's *Herball* (1597)

Thyme vinegar
Pick enough fresh **thyme** stems to fill a jar (use at least 464g or 1lb size); crush the herb in a mortar. Put into the jar and cover with a wine, cider or fruit **vinegar**. Keep closed jar in a sunny spot for at least a month, then strain off the vinegar.

The vinegar is good for headaches (rubbed onto temples and swallowed in small amounts), as a general antiseptic and for cleaning kitchen surfaces.

Thyme cough syrup
Mix 2 parts dried **thyme**, 1 part **fennel**, 1 part **licorice** and ½ part **poppy seed.**

Bring these to a boil in a pan of water, then cover and simmer for 20 minutes. Strain off the herbs and continue simmering until the liquid is reduced by at least a half and a syrup has formed.

Use for sore throat, deep coughs or asthma.

Za'atar
This is the Arabic for wild thyme (and related species), and also the name of a classic Middle Eastern spicy paste or condiment. Our simplified take on it follows:

2 parts **thyme** (fresh or dried leaf), 1 part **coriander seeds**, 1 part roasted **sesame seeds**, ½ part **rock salt.**

Pound ingredients in a mortar; add olive oil if needed to achieve a paste-like consistency. Serve with olive oil on pitta or other bread.

Thyme syrup
Warm a cupful of **honey** until it is runny, then add 3 teaspoons of crushed dried **thyme** (or 4 teaspoons of fresh thyme, chopped finely). Especially delicious if dried licorice is to hand and a tablespoon added.

This [list of attributes] *elevates the humble thyme into one of the finest remedies for the lungs.*
– Holmes (1989)

… a deep and powerful detoxifier.
– Wood (2008)

Thyme vinegar
• headaches
• colds
• fevers
• antiseptic
• sore throat

Thyme cough syrup
• colds
• fevers
• antiseptic
• sore throat
• asthma

Za'atar
• colds
• fevers
• antiseptic

Thyme syrup
• colds
• sore throats
• swollen glands

Turmeric *Curcuma longa*

English saffron, Haldi (Hindi), **Haridra** (Sanskrit), **Jiang huang** (Chinese medicine)

Turmeric root powder is a kitchen staple for adding colour and flavour to curries, rice and pickles, and a good natural orange–yellow dye. It also has a wealth of medicinal benefits, known in India and China for millennia, and which are coming to wider attention in the West, along with exciting research into potential new treatments. We rate turmeric as one of the principal kitchen medicines.

**Zingiberaceae
Ginger family**

Description: Perennial to 90cm (30in), with short stems, folded-over lanceolate leaves, a nubby brown rhizome with yellow–orange interior.

Distribution: Native to S and SE Asia, now cultivated all over tropical Asia.

Related species: *Curcuma aromatica* (wild turmeric), *C. amada* (mango ginger) and *C. zedoaria* (zedoary) are all used medicinally in India and China.

Parts used: Rhizomes.

... a vegetable which has all the properties of true saffron, as well the smell as the colour, and yet it is not really saffron.
– Marco Polo (1280)

Turmeric is a relative of ginger and is native to India and South-east Asia, requiring hot summer growing conditions. It is a smallish perennial plant, whose rhizomes (underground stems rather than roots) are crushed to make the familiar orange–yellow powder. Both the central bulbous and offshoot 'finger' rhizomes are used, and have a characteristic peppery, bitter taste and aroma.

India dominates the world trade in turmeric, and its use in the kitchen has followed Indian emigrants as they settle all over the world. It arrived later in the West than many other traded spices, and in 1280 Marco Polo was among the first to see it in China. He compared it to saffron in properties, smell and colour (though saffron is from a crocus).

The name stuck, and in French turmeric is *safran d'Inde*. Parkinson (1640) uses 'turmeric' but also an old Latin term, *Crocus indicus*, which suggests that the comparison persisted.

Turmeric is a standard ingredient of masala (cooking spice) mixes, an indispensable element of curries and a colourant for rice, pickles and chutneys. It also has a commercial use as a preservative in cheeses, cereals and yogurt, and even adds a yellow punch to the mustard used in American hot dogs.

Turmeric makes a fast natural dye (it is often the 'saffron' of Buddhist monks' robes), and has a central role in Hindu and Sikh marriage ceremonies, and cosmetic uses.

As an experiment for this book Julie tried a turmeric paste to tint her hair, which promptly went sea-green! It easily stains fingers and clothes, so treat carefully.

Fresh turmeric is less warming than the dried spice, and harder to find – try an Indian grocery or Oriental market.

Use turmeric for...
Turmeric has been known in Ayurvedic medicine for at least

four thousand years, and in Chinese medicine for almost as long. It is a traditional treatment for jaundice in both traditions, and used to stimulate the flow of blood and bile, while also helping to dissolve and prevent gallstones. It was once used in treating diabetes.

In Ayurveda it is seen as a blood 'purifier', and as a liver herb, which clears toxins. It is an effective skin cleanser and good for cataracts and conjunctivitis, along with a supplementary tonic effect on the gastrointestinal system and the lungs.

It is also used in India to regulate menstruation, and a poultice is applied for mastitis. It is a trusted external treatment for aching joints and tendons, and skin inflammations or wounds, combining its anti-inflammatory and antibacterial qualities.

Turmeric is also known as a yogic herb, for strengthening ligaments and purifying the inner channels or chakras.

In Chinese medicine it has been used in a similar range of treatments based on 'stagnant *qi*'.

In folk medicine terms, turmeric's antiseptic qualities are well recognised, and in Indian homes a cut or small bleeds will often be treated by covering with a pinch of haldi, the Hindi name for turmeric. The American manufacturer of BandAid™

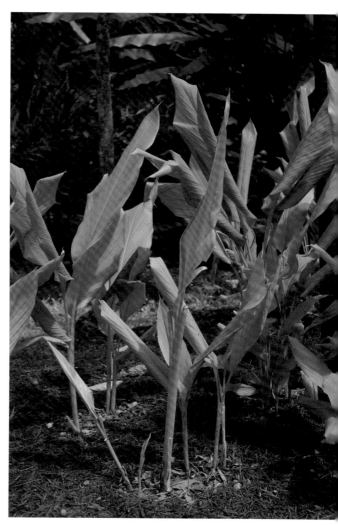

now produces a turmeric plaster specifically for export to India.

Another home remedy in India that will work equally well anywhere is 'golden milk', an old Ayurvedic cure-all and family standby. Turmeric boiled in water is also used to make a paste, which can be mixed with honey and swallowed like a pill or used externally. The turmeric paste can be stored in the fridge for a

Young turmeric shoots, Singapore, December

If I had hepatitis, I would add more turmeric to my cooking. – Duke (1997)

Turmeric helps to promote 'sweet' intestines by reducing pathogenic bacteria and destroying ama [toxins]. – Pole (2006)

few days. Drink golden milk for reducing the pain and stiffness of arthritis and rheumatism (turmeric is a wonderful anti-inflammatory), and as a tonic for poor digestion; externally you can use the paste for skin conditions, especially psoriasis, and for rubbing on aching joints.

Joe and Teresa Graedon report how one American who had suffered from psoriasis for 25 years and had tried every medical intervention, at great personal cost and frustration, began to sprinkle a heaped tablespoon of turmeric powder on his morning cereal. In 10 days the itching and bleeding stopped; after eight weeks the problems on his legs and thighs cleared up; and after five months the condition was cured.

It was not a placebo effect, the Graedons suggest, as someone else's potbellied pig was about to

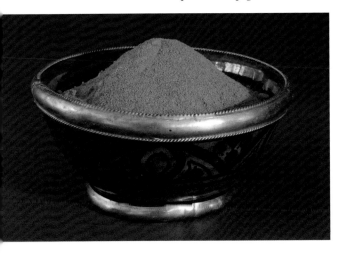

be put down when nothing could improve its disc problem. Taking turmeric as curcumin pills got the pig back to full health.

Such stories are individual and anecdotal, of course, but what is really exciting about turmeric is a mass of recent scientific research that supports many of the older medicinal claims but also adds promising new ones.

This signifies a drastic change in attitudes towards turmeric. Writing in 1931, and speaking for western herbalism of the time, Mrs Grieve could only find this to say:

Turmeric is a mild aromatic stimulant seldom used in medicine except as a colouring. It was once a cure for jaundice. Its chief use is in the manufacture of curry powders.

Now there are many hundreds of articles online on PubMed, the website of the US National Library of Medicine and the National Institutes of Health, examining a seemingly unlimited beneficial potential for curcumin, the yellow-coloured pigment of turmeric (see box). The overall trend of such research is transiting from successful animal and in vitro studies to first-stage human trials (small groups) and full-scale clinical trials for some conditions.

The interesting thing here is that curcumin – called 'Indian solid gold' by one leading pharmacological researcher in the States, Dr B.B. Aggarwal – cannot be patented. A US patent was actually granted in 1995, but this was overturned on appeal, opponents successfully showing traditional and broad-acting use for turmeric and curcumin.

We mention this because it serves to indicate that curcumin must be deeply promising, as without patents pharmaceutical companies are reluctant to fund very costly full human trials. Turmeric is perhaps just too broad and complementary to fit an easy pharmaceutical mould. Ayurvedic doctors – and Indian mothers – would probably say, 'ah, at last you are catching up!'

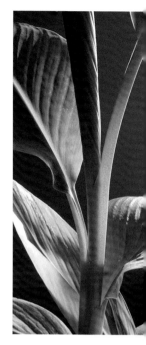

Golden milk

This is a traditional Indian formula to boost the immune system, and is particularly beneficial for older people. With sweet almond oil, it also helps keep the joints supple.

Add ½ to 1 teaspoonful **turmeric** powder to ½ cup **water** in a small saucepan. Simmer for about 5 minutes, then add 1 cup of **milk** (or almond milk). Add a pinch of **black pepper** to increase absorption. Add between a teaspoon and 2 tablespoons of **sweet almond oil**. Bring just to the boiling point, then remove from heat. Add **honey** to taste, and drink hot. If you are taking it for your joints, drink a cup daily, using the higher amount of almond oil.

Golden electuary

Mix **turmeric** powder into **honey** to make a paste.

Use externally on cuts and wounds; internally take 1 teaspoonful several times a day for fevers. Can be eaten as is, or try it blended in a cup of warm water with lime juice, or in a cooling fruit smoothie.

Golden milk
- boosts immunity
- convalescence
- old age
- joint health

Golden electuary
- cuts
- wounds
- fevers
- inflammation

Indian solid gold: curcumin

The active pigment in turmeric is curcumin, sometimes called turmeric yellow. Among research developments being reported are:

- curcumin interferes with replication of HIV, *Herpes simplex* and malarial cells, without harming the body's healthy cells;
- it boosts the auto-immune response in older people;
- it blocks signalling pathways that lead to Alzheimer's disease;
- it intervenes in the growth of certain cancer cells and tumours, and helps make chemotherapy treatments more effective (especially in colon and skin cancers);
- it enhances beneficial effects of radiation treatment, apparently by preventing tumour cells developing radiation resistance;
- it lowers total cholesterol, preventing functioning of LDL ('bad') cholesterol while also raising HDL ('good') cholesterol, increasing the blood-thinning capacity. This may benefit people with atherosclerosis or those at risk of stoke or heart attacks;
- it binds some heavy metals, including lead, and also iron and copper.

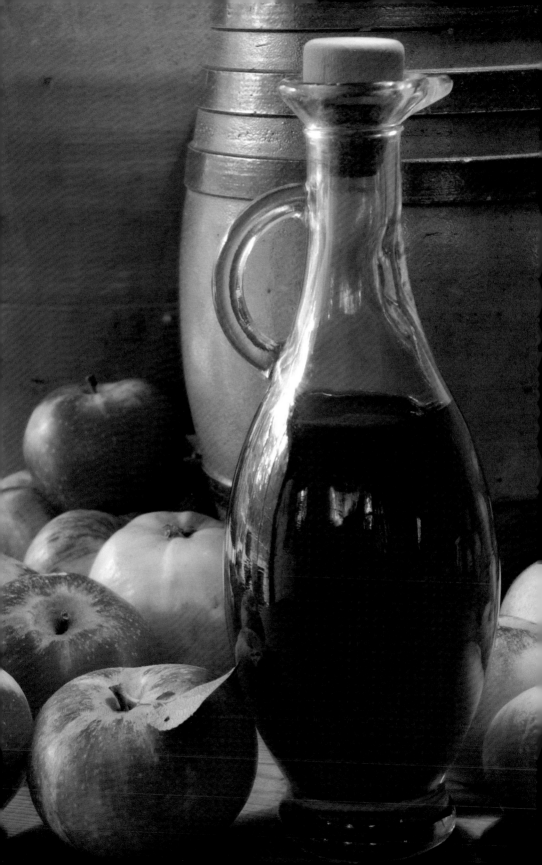

Vinegar Acetic acid

In addition to its role in cooking and as a preservative, vinegar is a ready cleaner for kitchen surfaces. It also earns its place as a natural and versatile home remedy, which is both inexpensive and safe to use. Externally, it combats fungal infections of the skin and head, and is effective for burns and sunburn. Internally, taken as apple cider vinegar, it is said to relieve many ills and be an excellent healthy morning drink.

The origins of vinegar are not known, but as its formation is a natural process it must have been discovered rather than invented. In any alcoholic liquid exposed to air the bacteria present will oxidise the alcohol into acetic acid, the chemical name for vinegar.

This process was once a problem for wine storage, as air entering any barrel or bottle would convert the alcohol into vinegar. Indeed, the very name 'vinegar' is from old French *vin* and *aigre*, meaning 'sharp wine'.

Cork plugs proved better than previous methods of using clay and wax or rags to stopper vessels, the cork expanding to fit any size of hole and being reusable.

All the same, a fermented wine is not necessarily good vinegar. The finest vinegars are slow-matured, and in the case of a true balsamic vinegar from Modena or Reggio in Italy the ageing process may take decades.

In the kitchen, vinegar is traditionally used in salad dressings, sauces and in pickles, and as a preservative for fruits, vegetables and herbs. We'd love to invite you round to try our delicious home-made raspberry vinegar!

Use vinegar for...

Vinegar is a weak acid based on bacterial fermentation. As such it readily destroys fungal and yeast infections on the skin, such as athlete's foot and thrush. Spray vinegar in your shoes if you suffer from fungal foot infections.

Used externally, it neutralises the venom of wasp stings, is cooling and soothing for burns and sunburn, and also relieves dandruff. A cold vinegar compress draws heat from swellings, and was applied to the feet in fevers.

If you know your nursery rhymes, in 'Jack and Jill', Jack 'went to bed to mend his head with vinegar and brown paper' – an eighteenth-century vinegar compress.

Source: Almost any plant material can be used to make alcohol, with the fermentation of yeast turning sugars to alcohol. Vinegar is a secondary fermentation by bacteria, in the presence of air, converting the alcohol to acetic acid. The most common vinegars are made from cider, wine, malt or rice-based drinks. There is also distilled white or spirit vinegar, which is much harsher.

Vinegar might just be one of the most versatile home remedies there is. ... As for most home remedies, there is little, if any, scientific research to back up the claims. Then again, vinegar is inexpensive, and the likelihood of side effects is low. After all, we use it in salads, how dangerous can it be?
– Graedon & Graedon (2006)

[Vinegar is] *sharpe and penetrating, and very usefull in scabbes, itches, tetters, ring-wormes, and fretting and creeping ulcers, to correct their malignancy, and extirpate their corroding quality.*
– Parkinson (1640)

'Tis cutting, digestive, and opening; 'tis very good to extinguish the heat of Choler, and Thirst, strengthens the Gums, excites the Appetite, removes Obstructions, aids Digestion, and is good for hot and moist Stomachs, weakens the Blood, the Choler, and resists Putrefaction; therefore in the time of the Plague, many used it, to preserve themselves.
– Chamberlayne (1689)

Vinegar added to a bath or to rinses helps maintain a healthy pH balance and helps destroy yeast infections while protecting the skin. With warm water as a hair rinse, it leaves hair shiny and clean.

In 1958 apple cider vinegar had its day in the sun with publication of the book *Folk Medicine* by Dr DC Jarvis (1881–1966). This popular, influential work, based on Vermont home medicine, argues for cider vinegar in warm water every morning as the cure for most ills.

John Chamberlayne (1689) disagreed: 'You must not use it at Breakfast, and always moderately.' Vinegar was best with raisins or anise or fennel; it 'is not good for Ladies, for it causes wrinkles, &c.'

The late Doctor James Malone's receipt for a cold
An early nineteenth-century English remedy

'Take a large teacupfull of Linseed, two pennyworth of Stick Liquorice, and a quarter of a pound of Jar raisins—put these into 2 quarts of soft water and let it simmer over a slow fire till it is reduced to one, then add to it a ¼ of a pound of brown sugar candy, a tablespoonful of old Rum and a tablespoonful of the best white wine vinegar or Lemon juice. Drink half a pint going to bed and take a little when the cough is troublesome.

'This Receipt generally cures the worst of colds in two or three days and if taken in time may be almost said to be an infallible remedy—It is a most sovereign and balsamic cordial to the lungs, without the opening qualities which endanger fresh colds on going out—It has been known to cure colds that have been almost settled in Consumption in less than three weeks.'

Sage and vinegar fomentation
Put a small bunch of fresh **sage leaves** in a blender with half a cup of **vinegar** (and half cup **hot water**), and blend until green. Warm in a saucepan until hot but not boiling. Strain the liquid into a small bowl, and soak cotton balls or a piece of gauze in the liquid. Apply hot to sprains and bruises, cover with a piece of cling-film or wax paper then a towel, and keep hot with a hot water bottle or heating pad. Leave on for an hour or until swelling has subsided.

Vinegar baths
A daily 20 minute bath in hot water 38°C (100°F) and cider vinegar (add 1 cup to the bath) can cleanse the body of acid residues. Vinegar baths are an additional therapy for fungal skin diseases and for treating vaginitis. Vinegar baths can be safely taken over a six-week period.

Sage & vinegar fomentation
- bruises
- sprains

Vinegar baths
- dry skin
- fungal infections
- vaginitis

Water

Water is essential for life, and comprises the largest single component of our body, at 45–75% of our total weight. Water is a solvent and a lubricant, which enables internal chemical reactions and helps maintain a stable body temperature. Let us demystify the science of water by looking at how its qualities are the basis for hydrotherapy and other simple home treatments.

Britain is blessed in having plenty of water. To Julie it is a luxury, as she has lived in several arid countries where rain is rare and precious. English friends think she is mad for loving the sound of rain on the tiles! As the vagaries of climate change create severe drought in so many marginal arid regions, places with regular rain should rejoice, not grouse.

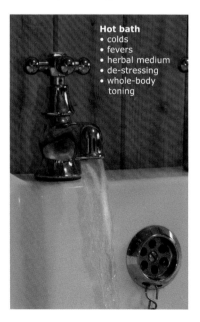

Hot bath
- colds
- fevers
- herbal medium
- de-stressing
- whole-body toning

So, what does all this have to do with health? Besides the obvious fact that we all need water to drink to stay alive, and our bodies are more water than anything else, water has valuable therapeutic properties.

One of these is its high specific heat, which technically speaking is the amount of heat per unit mass required to raise the temperature by one degree Celsius. The specific heat of water is 1 calorie per gram per degree Celsius, which is higher than any other common substance. What this means is that water 'holds' a lot of heat, and as a result plays a vital role in our own temperature regulation.

Before your eyes glaze over, in a practical sense this means that hot water contains more heat than most other substances at the same temperature, which makes it ideal at heating us up. In terms of your own inner temperature, taking a moderately hot bath is the best way to warm yourself if you are chilled, and we all appreciate hot-water bottles on chilly winter nights.

Description: Water has the chemical formula H_2O.

Properties: Water has a high specific heat of 1 calorie/gram °C = 4.186 joule/gram °C.

Water freezes at 0°C (32°F), and boils at 100°C (212 °F) at sea level.

At high altitudes, with a decrease in atmospheric pressure, water boils at a lower temperature. Elevation, however, has little effect on the freezing point.

There must be quite a few things that a hot bath won't cure, but I don't know many of them.
– Sylvia Plath (1963)

Neutral bath
33.5°C–35.6°C
• stress
• tension
• insomnia
• tight muscles
• colds

Cold shower
• invigorating
• warming
• closes pores

When you heat water in a kettle or on the stove, it absorbs heat until it reaches boiling point and changes from a liquid to a gas. During the transition, the temperature remains constant until the change is completed. So at sea level with one atmosphere of pressure, water always boils at 100°C.

Conversely, cold water absorbs heat from our bodies quickly as it takes a lot of heat to warm it up.

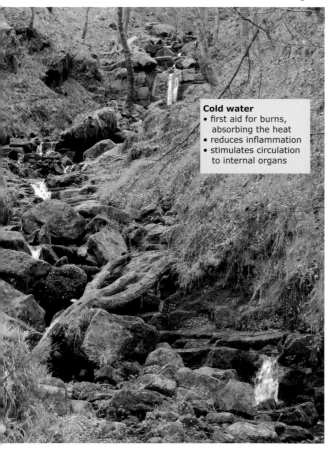

Cold water
• first aid for burns, absorbing the heat
• reduces inflammation
• stimulates circulation to internal organs

So, first aid for burns is to hold the affected area under cool running water immediately. Continue for 10–15 minutes or until the pain subsides. Ice absorbs heat until it reaches its melting point of 0°C, and remains at that temperature until it all liquefies.

Hydrotherapy (water therapy) is the therapeutic use of water at different temperatures to revitalise, maintain and restore health. Treatment options include hot springs, saunas, vapour, steam, foot and sitz baths, cold and hot water compresses and ice packs.

Cold water is stimulating as it causes superficial blood vessels to constrict, sending the blood deeper into the body to the internal organs. Hot water is relaxing, causes blood vessels to dilate, and removes wastes from body tissues. Alternating hot and cold water also improves elimination, decreases inflammation and stimulates circulation.

Bath water kept at body temperature has a marked relaxing and sedative effect on the nervous system, benefiting various stressed states. Used for short periods, the neutral bath is a self-help measure that will sedate the nervous system. Keep the water temperature between 33.5° and 35.6°C with a bath thermometer, and take care to ensure that the bathroom is also kept warm.

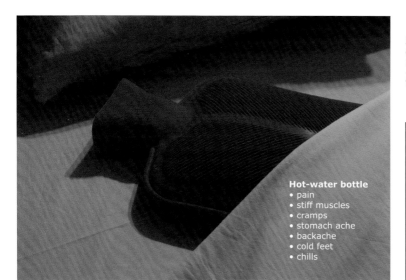

Even the Archbishop of Canterbury is 65% water.
– Haldane (early/mid-twentieth century)

Hot-water bottle
- pain
- stiff muscles
- cramps
- stomach ache
- backache
- cold feet
- chills

Our water world
Measuring the proportion of water as a **percentage of body weight**, infants have the highest level, up to 75%, but this decreases with age. Because fat tissue contains almost no water, fat people have a smaller proportion of water than slim people. A normal adult male is about 60% water by weight, while women generally have more subcutaneous fat, and average 55% water.

Ingested liquids and foods make up about 2300ml of our **water intake** a day – the so-called pre-formed water. Another source is metabolic water, at about 200ml a day, the product of our cellular-level respiration.

At the other side of the balance, we **eliminate water** through the urine (about 1500ml a day); the skin (about 400ml via evaporation and around 200ml as sweat); the lungs (exhaling about 300ml); and the faeces (excreting about 100ml). Menstruation also involves water loss.

Half an hour of immersion in a body-temperature bath has a sedative, even soporific, effect. It does not strain the heart, circulation or nervous system and achieves muscular relaxation and expansion of the blood vessels. The bath can be used in conjunction with other methods of relaxation, such as breathing techniques and meditation, to make it an even more effective way of wiping out stress. Use daily if you find it helpful.

Steam baths and saunas encourage sweating, opening the pores and increasing elimination through the skin. Just as these treatments are traditionally followed by plunging in cold water or rolling in the snow to close the pores again, it's a good idea to follow a long hot bath with a quick cold shower. Admit it, a cold shower is stimulating, refreshing and energising – it helps you feel warmer later because closing the pores prevents further heat loss through the skin, and stimulates the body to produce heat to counteract the cold.

How much water do you need to drink? Most of us don't drink enough, although drinking too much puts extra work on the kidneys and can deplete our electrolytes. Quantities depend on what we are eating: a diet of salted meat and dry biscuits makes you thirstier than fruit and salads, or soup. How much you are sweating from exercise or hot weather has an impact, as does the humidity of the air. In an arid environment like a desert, an airliner or a centrally heated office, you lose moisture at each breath and need to replenish by drinking water plentifully.

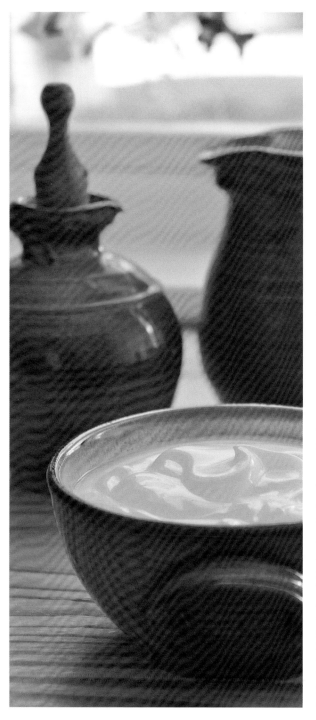

Yogurt

Yogurt is a traditional fermented milk product. It is easier to digest than milk, and its live bacterial cultures are beneficial to our health in many ways. Yogurt is particularly useful after antibiotic treatment, and is effective against thrush.

Yogurt and other fermented milk products are dietary staples of pastoral peoples around the world, and have probably been a part of the human diet since the first animals were domesticated and milked.

Yogurt is eaten fresh (it stores much better than milk) and goes into a variety of cheeses and drinks. In Lebanon, *lebne* is made by straining yogurt and adding salt, shaped into balls, dried and stored in olive oil.

Yogurt is much easier to digest than milk for people with lactose intolerance, as the lactose has been broken down by the bacterial fermentation. White Europeans can usually digest lactose, but many other peoples, especially from Africa and Asia, can lose the ability to digest milk once they grow up. If you are dairy intolerant, try a non-dairy version such as coconut yogurt.

The character of a yogurt will depend on many factors, primarily the type of milk and the cultures used. Other micro-organisms present will give different characteristics. Buffalo milk yogurt is sweet and mild, whereas yogurt made with skimmed cow milk is much more thin and sour. Traditionally yogurts were made using whole milk that was fresh, unpasteurised and unhomogenised.

It is particularly helpful to eat yogurt after antibiotic treatment, especially broad-spectrum antibiotics, which kill off much of our beneficial gut bacteria. A healthy gut flora is important not only for good digestion, which benefits health as a whole, but is vital for continued immunity.

Science supports the benefits of eating yogurt, and it is being trialled in NHS hospitals to help reduce *Clostridium difficile* infection caused by antibiotic use.

Applying yogurt brings quick relief to the itching of vaginal and vulval thrush infections and to the equivalent infection in men. If the infection is recurrent, both partners need to be treated. The yogurt can be mixed with warm water and turmeric powder as a douche and a 'willy wash'. The same mixture works for fungal skin infections such as ringworm.

Yogurt makes an effective moisturising and toning face mask, which restores the skin's natural protective acidity. Apply, leave a few minutes, then rinse off.

Source: The bacteria that produce yogurt ferment milk lactose into lactic acid, which gives yogurt its characteristic sour taste.

Yogurt can be made from any milk: cow, goat, sheep, camel, water buffalo, mare and dri (yak) are the best-known. Various non-dairy yogurts are also available, made using live cultures and soy, coconut or other nutmilks.

The bacteria vary depending on where the yogurt is made, but much commercial yogurt is cultured with strains of *Lactobacillus bulgaricus* and *Streptococcus thermophilus*, which orginated in Turkey and the Balkans.

Similar products: An ancient cultured milk from the Caucasus, kefir, contains the same bacteria as yogurts but in addition has a yeast, *Saccharomyces kefir*, which causes it to fizz and gives it a slight alcohol content.

Yogurt eaten
- after antibiotics
- digestion
- immunity
- antibiotic-associated diarrhoea
- oral thrush

External use
- vaginal thrush
- oral thrush
- itchy skin

Making your own yogurt

Fresh home-made yogurt is as good as many more expensive pro- bi- otic products on the market, and is easy to make. You'll find many variations in recipes, but this is a simple one to get you going.

You'll need a couple of tablespoons of bought **live yogurt** as your starter. Let this warm up to room temperature while you get the milk ready. Gently heat your **milk** in a clean pan until it starts to foam – you can do this over a pan of water so that it doesn't burn on the bottom, or just keep an eye on it as it heats. Allow it to cool until it feels warm to the finger, before adding your culture and stirring it in. If you have a thermometer, check the temperature, as anything over 55°C (130°F) will kill the culture.

The bacteria that make yogurt want warmth, and will be inactive under 37°C (98°F), so you need to keep your culture warm while it ferments. One of the easiest ways is to pour it into a thermos flask and leave overnight. Your yogurt will be ready in the morning! Before you use it, set aside a small amount in a clean jar to keep in the fridge as your starter for the next batch.

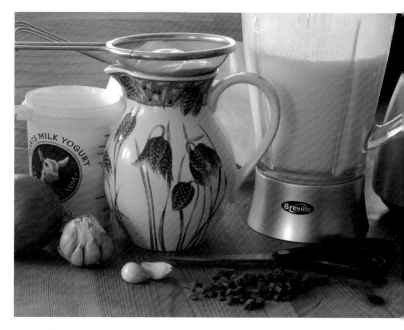

Tzadziki

A cooling dip. If using ordinary **yogurt**, spoon it into a fine strainer or a sieve lined with muslin or cheesecloth. Let it drip until it is nice and thick. Save the liquid for use in cooking. If you want to shortcut this step, buy Greek yogurt, which has already been strained.

Into a cup of strained yogurt, stir 1 to 2 teaspoons minced **garlic** and a tablespoon of chopped **chives**. **Salt** to taste. Let it sit for an hour or more at room temperature to allow the flavours to blend.

Traditional recipes often include cucumber, which our version omits, and some people add dill leaf and mint leaf. Finely minced raw onion can also be used, and black pepper or grated lemon zest added.

Serve as a dip with pitta bread or as a sauce.

Lassi

Use 1 cup each of **yogurt** and **water** to make this Indian favourite.
For sweet lassi, blend with a little brown sugar or maple syrup to taste.
For salt lassi, add ½ teaspoon salt and 1 teaspoon cumin seed, or to taste.
For mango lassi, add the flesh of a mango.

Add fresh ginger to either sweet or salty lassi. Cilantro leaves go well with salt lassi. Cardamom powder adds another level to sweet lassi.

Quick reference by ailment

Ailments are listed alphabetically. Remedies are listed in order of our preference, or otherwise aphabetically.

Aches & pains
Hot pain-relieving oil: p53
Clove and black pepper ointment: p37
Cabbage: p41
Hot healing oil: p103
Hot-water bottle: p185
Mustard foot bath (aching legs and feet): p114

Acne
Gentle liver cleanse: p125
Lemon juice: use as a lotion. p107
Sage tea: use as a wash for oily skin. p159

Age spots (liver spots)
Lemon juice: rub the spots with a slice of lemon twice a day. p107
Cilantro & lemon lotion: p75
Banana peel: rub the spots with the inner side of fresh peel twice a day. p17
Gentle liver cleanse: p125

Allergies
Three spice powder: half a teaspoonful mixed with a little local honey three times a day or as often as needed. p9

Anaemia
Beetroot: p27
Parsley: eat plenty on a regular basis. p136
Pineapple: p145

Anxiety
Nutmeg: p117

Appetite, poor
Orange & cardamom bitters: p132
Aniseed: p8
Coconut chutney: p67
Coriander: hippocras, dukka. p75

Arthritis
Celery and celery seed: eat celery regularly; take ½ teaspoon celery seed daily. p48
Cabbage poultice: to cool inflamed joints. p41
Hot pain-relieving oil: topical pain relief. p53
Hot healing oil: p103
Oxymel: p106
Parsley root decoction: p139

Asthma
Aniseed tea: drink the tea & inhale the vapour. p8
Onion poultice: helps loosen a tight chest. p129

Athlete's foot
Turmeric powder: applied twice daily. p176
Cornflour: as a foot powder. p79
Coconut anti-fungal ointment: p67

Backache
Hot pain-relieving oil: p53
Hot healing oil: p103
Hot water-bottle: the gentle heat helps relax muscles. p185

Bee stings
Bicarb paste: p31

Bladder problems
Barley water: p21
Cornsilk tea: p79

Bleeding
Chilli powder: sprinkle on the cut. p53
Pressure: apply pressure to the wound to stop bleeding.
Lemon: sprinkle the cut with lemon juice. p107

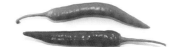

Bloating after eating

Eating: make sure you are relaxed when you eat, and chew your food well. Bloating may be a sign of a food intolerance.
Fennel: chew a few seeds after eating. p88
Pineapple: p145
Orange & cardamom bitters: take a teaspoonful 10 or 15 minutes before eating, or take after a meal. p132

Blood pressure

Cinnamon decoction: p61

Blood sugar imbalances

Eating: eat smaller meals more often. Don't miss meals. Avoid sugar and other high glycaemic-index foods.
Exercise: reduces insulin resistance.
Fenugreek tea: p93
Cinnamon: p58
Barley soup: p21
Banana almond smoothie (low blood sugar): p17

Boils

Cabbage: poultice. p41
Ginger poultice: p103
Water: apply a cloth dipped in hot water, as hot as you can stand, reheating as needed.

Breast feeding (lactation)

Sore breasts:
Cabbage: put a leaf inside your bra. p38
To increase milk production:
Fennel seed: p88
Fenugreek: p93
To dry up milk:
Sage: drink cold sage tea. p156
Parsley: eat lots of fresh parsley. p136

Breath, bad

Parsley: chew some fresh parsley. p136
Cardamom: chew a pod or two. p42
Allspice: chew a fruit, or make a tea. p2
Tooth cleaning powder: p31
Sage tooth powder: p159

Bronchitis

Lemon & sage drink: p109
Onion poultice: p129
Oregano tincture: p135

Bruises

Pineapple poultice: p145
Rosemary: p152
Sage & vinegar fomentation: p182

Burns

Water: First aid: hold the burned area under cold water for ten minutes. p183
Banana peel: p16
Cling-film: the perfect dressing for more serious burns before you go to A&E. Protects without sticking.
Onion: use the thin transparent film between onion layers as a protective dressing. p126

Catarrh

Avoid dairy products, as they increase mucus.
Chillies: p50
Three spice powder: p9

Chapped skin

Olive oil: p122
Carrot oil: p47
Coconut oil: p65
Ghee: p37

Chicken pox

Bicarb bath: p31

Chilblains

Clove & black pepper ointment: p37
Hot pain-relieving oil: p53
Ginger tea: to improve circulation. p103
Mustard foot bath: p114

Cholesterol, high

Barley soup: p21
Cinnamon tincture: p61
Fenugreek tea: p93

Onions: eat onions, leeks or garlic regularly.

Circulation
Ginger tea: p103
Garlic: p96
Onions: p126
Chocolate: p 57
Allspice tea: p4
Cold-banishing soup: p53
Hippocras: p75
Mulligatawny soup: p143
Quatre épices: p143
Rosemary: tea or wine. p155

Cold feet
Clove & black pepper ointment: p37
Hot pain-relieving oil: p53
Mustard foot bath: p114

Colds
Cold-banishing soup: p53
Fenugreek tea: p93
Garlic: p99
Ginger: tea, ginger and onion soup, bath. p103
Hippocras: p75
Lemon: with sage, or ginger. p109
Aniseed: three spice powder and aniseed tea with thyme. p9
Mulligatawny soup: p143
Mustard foot bath: p114
Neutral bath: p184
Quatre épices: p143
Thyme: vinegar, cough syrup. p175

Colic
Dill: p87
Aniseed & thyme tea: p9

Colitis
Almond milk: p7
Barley soup: p21

Concentration
Basil tea: p25
Rosemary tea: p155
Oregano tea: p135

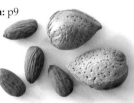

Constipation
Figs: eat a few figs, or take fig syrup. p95
Prunes: eat a few dried or stewed prunes, or drink prune juice.
Coffee: drinking a cup of strong coffee has an immediate laxative effect, unless you are a heavy coffee drinker. p68
Almond milk: p7
Barley soup: p21

Convalescence
Apple: grated with ginger, sauce. p13
Arrowroot pudding: p15
Barley: soup, barley water. p21
Cardamom: p45
Golden milk: p179
Honey butter: p36
Kichri: p151
Oats: p118
Rice milk: p151
Rosemary: tea or wine. p155

Coughs
Thyme cough syrup: p175
Almond milk (dry cough): p7
Aniseed & thyme tea: p9
Barley water: for dry cough. p21
Cardamom: electuary, syrup. p45
Cold-banishing soup: p53
Garlic: p96
Garlic honey: p99
Marjoram conserve: p135
Onion poultice: p129
Oregano: tea or tincture. p135
Pepper: mulligatawny soup, quatre épices. p143

Cramps
Banana almond smoothie: p17
Hot-water bottle (menstrual cramps): p185

Cuts and grazes
Cabbage poultice: p41
Garlic honey: p99
Golden electuary: p179
Honey: p104
Salt: p163

Cystitis
Parsley: eat lots of parsley or make parsley tea, jelly or root decoction. p139
Barley water: p21
Blueberries: p33
Cranberry: p80
Cornsilk tea: p79

Dandruff
Coconut oil scalp conditioner: p67
Lemon: add lemon juice to your hair rinse. p107
Rosemary scalp conditioner: p155
Sage vinegar: p159
Vinegar: add vinegar to your hair rinse. p180

Dehydration
Oral rehydration solution: p167
Corpse reviver: p31
Jaljeera: p84
Nimbu lemonade: p109

Depression, mild
Basil tea: p25
Oregano tea: p135
Rosemary: p152

Diarrhoea
Arrowroot pudding: p15
Corpse reviver: p31
Grated apple and ginger: p13
Oral rehydration solution: p167
From antibiotics:
Yogurt: p187

Digestive problems
Because nearly all herbs and spices found in the kitchen help digestion, this is only a partial list of our top recommendations.
Orange & cardamom bitters: p132
Aniseed: p8
Dill: gas and griping pains. p85
Fennel: gas and griping pains. p88
Coriander: dukka, hippocras. p75
Cumin: p84
Ginger: nausea, gas and griping. p100
Allspice: p2

Apple: p13
Cardamom: p42
Carrot lassi: p47
Cinnamon tincture: p61
Coconut chutney: p67
Fenugreek: p93
Masala chai: p172
Oregano: p133
Pepper: p140
Pineapple: p144

Dry skin
Ghee: p37
Carrot oil: p47
Cilantro & lemon lotion: p75

Ear ache
Garlic in olive oil: pp122 and 96

Eczema
Hemp seed oil: take 1 teaspoonful with food three times a day, or ½ teaspoonful for children.
Gentle liver cleanse: p125
Carrot oil: p47
Oat bath: p121

Energy
Banana almond smoothie: p17
Barley water & soup: p21
Honey butter: p36
Elachi energiser: p45

Eyes
Blueberries: p33
Eye refresher: p172
Gentle liver cleanse: p125
Parsley tea eyebath: p139
Salt water eyebath: p163

Fevers
Cinnamon: p61
Garlic: p99
Ginger: p100
Golden electuary: p179
Thyme vinegar: p175

Flatulence and gas
Aniseed: p8
Allspice tea: p4
Cumin tea: p84
Digestive tea: p84
Dill: p85
Fennel: p88

'Flu
Cinnamon tincture: p61
Cold-banishing soup: p53
Four thieves vinegar: p99
Garlic honey: p99
Lemon & ginger tea: p109

Fluid retention (oedema)
Cornsilk tea: p79
Parsley root decoction: p139
Pumpkin seeds: p149

Foggy head
Clove & oat scrub: p64
Oregano: tea or tincture. p135
Gentle liver cleanse: p125

Freckles
Cilantro & lemon lotion: p75

Fungal infections
Arrowroot: as a powder. p15
Cornflour: as a powder. p79
Turmeric powder: applied twice daily. p176
Coconut anti-fungal ointment: p67
Foot powder: p79

Gout
Celery: p48

Gum problems
Allspice mouthwash: p4
Sage tooth powder: p159

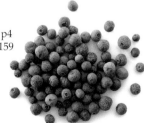

Hair
Arrowroot: as a dry shampoo. p15
Cornflour: as a dry shampoo. p79
Scalp conditioner: p67
Sage vinegar: p159

Hangover
Clove scrub: p64
Gentle liver cleanse: p125
Water: drink plenty. p183

Hayfever
Three spice powder: take half teaspoonful mixed with a little local honey three times daily as needed. p9

Headache
Basil tea: p25
Coffee: while coffee can cause headaches, it can also alleviate them (caffeine is often added to aspirin tablets). p68
Coriander tea: p75
Oregano tea or tincture: p135
Rosemary tea: p155
Thyme vinegar: p175

Heart & circulation
Chilli: p50
Ginger: p100
Garlic: p96
Turmeric: p176

Hiccups
Water: drink a glass of water from the far side of the glass, holding your fingers in your ears. It sounds weird, but it's the one method we've found that works better than anything else.

Hoarseness
Cardamom syrup: p45
Three spice powder: mix with honey. p9

Hot flushes/flashes
Water: drink a glass of cool water at the first sign of ash.
Sage tea: drink cold. p159

Immunity
Barley soup: p21
Beetroot juice: p27
Golden milk: p179
Immune-boosting soup: p111
Yogurt: p187

Indigestion (dyspepsia)
Basil tea: p25
Digestive tea: p84
Pineapple: p145
Star anise tea: p165

Infections
Four thieves' vinegar: p99
Garlic: p99
Garlic butter: p36
Garlic honey: p99
Oregano tincture: p135
Thyme vinegar: p173

Inflammation
Cabbage: p41
Turmeric: p176

Insect bites and stings
Allspice paste: p4
Banana peel: rub the bite with the inside of a banana peel. p17
Bicarb paste: bee stings. p31
Vinegar: wasp stings. p180
Parsley: poultice of crushed parsley. p 136

Insomnia
Nutmeg: p115
Poppy seed electuary: p146
Water: neutral bath. p184

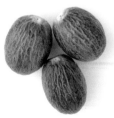

Irritable bowel syndrome (IBS)
Food intolerances: wheat and dairy are the most common causes of intolerances.
Almond milk: p7
Barley soup: p21
Coriander tea: p75
Fenugreek tea: p93

Itchy skin
Bicarb bath: p31
Carrot oil: p47
Oat bath: p121

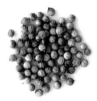

Jet lag
Clove & oat scrub: p64

Joints
Cabbage: hot, inflamed joints. p41
Clove and black pepper ointment: p37
Hot healing oil: p103
Hot pain-relieving oil: p53
Golden milk: p179

Lymphoedema
Cabbage poultice: p41

Mastitis
Cabbage poultice: p41
Hot pain-relieving oil: p53

Memory
Basil tea: p25
Rosemary tea: p155
Sage tea: p159

Menopausal symptoms
Allspice tea: p4
Sage tea: p159

Menstruation
Fenugreek tea: p93
Parsley, sage & rosemary tea: balances hormones.

Mouth and throat
Oregano tea: p135
Salt gargle: p163
Sage mouthwash: p159
Bicarbonate of soda: p31

Nappy rash (diaper rash)
Cornflour: as a powder. p79
Coconut oil: p65
Olive oil: p122

Nausea
Ginger tea: p103
Digestive tea: p84
Grated apple and ginger: p13

Nosebleeds
Ice water: apply as a compress at the back of the neck.

Period pain
Hot-water bottle: relaxes cramps. p 185
Ginger tea: p103

Pimples
Gentle liver cleanse: p125
Lemon juice: use as a lotion. p107
Sage tea: use as a wash for oily skin. p159

Prostate problems
Pumpkin seeds: eat 2 handfuls a day. p148
Cornsilk tea: p79
Cranberry: p80

Rashes
Bicarb bath: p31
Soda paste: p31
Oat bath: p121

Shingles
Chilli oil: p53
Bicarb bath: p31
Soda paste: p31

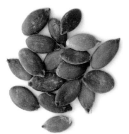

Sinus congestion
Horseradish: chew a teaspoonful of grated horseradish as needed.
Pepper: chew a few green peppercorns. p140
Star anise tea: p165

Skin problems
Bicarb bath: for itching. p31
Carrot oil: for dryness. p47
Gentle liver cleanse: p125
Hemp seed oil: eat 1 teaspoonful with food three times a day, or ½ teaspoonful for children
Oat bath: p121
Vinegar bath: p182

Sore throat
Cardamom: electuary & syrup. p45
Lemon and ginger: p109
Lemon and sage: p109
Marjoram conserve: p135
Pepper: chew a few green peppercorns. p140
Pineapple: p144
Salt gargle: p163
Thyme: vinegar, syrup, cough syrup. p175

Splinters
Sugar and soap poultice: p167
Cabbage poultice: p41
Onion poultice: p129

Sprains
Cold water: apply cold water or an ice pack.
Frozen peas: wrap a packet from the fridge in a towel and apply to the injury.
Hot pain-relieving oil: p53
Sage & vinegar fomentation: p182
Cabbage poultice: p41
Water: hot and cold soaks. p183

Stained teeth
Bicarbonate of soda: wet your finger or a cotton bud, dip into some bicarb, and polish your teeth with it. Rinse your mouth frequently with water.

Stress
Aztec cocoa: p57
Dill tea: p87
Nutmeg: p115
Rosemary tea: p155

Sunburn
Banana peel: p17
Bicarb bath: p31
Cabbage poultice: p41
Carrot oil: p47
Tea: apply cold tea bags or tea leaves. p168
Yogurt: use as a cooling lotion. p186

Teeth
Sage: mouthwash, tooth powder. p 159
Tooth cleaning powder: p31

Threadworm
Carrot: eat only grated carrot for a day. p46
Coconut: take a tablespoon of freshly ground coconut at breakfast, followed by a teaspoon of castor oil. p65
Garlic: eat 4 or 5 cloves raw garlic a day. p96
Pumpkin seed: paralyses the worms: eat a handful of seeds and follow with a laxative. p148
Thyme tea: take strong with lemon juice at breakfast for two weeks. p173

Thrush
Turmeric: turmeric powder in warm water. p176
Yogurt: p186
Vinegar: p180
Garlic: p96
Allspice: p2
Sage vinegar: p159

Toothache
Allspice: chew an allspice berry or pack the affected tooth with allspice powder. p2
Cloves: chew a clove as needed. p62
Ginger: chew a piece of fresh ginger. p100

Ulcers (stomach & duodenal)
Cabbage juice: p38

Urinary infections
Parsley: eat lots of parsley or make parsley tea, jelly or root decoction. p139
Barley water: p21
Blueberries: p33
Cranberry: p80
Cornsilk tea: p79

Vaginal dryness:
Fennel: tea, ointment. p91
Fenugreek tea. p93

Varicose & thread veins
Blueberries: p32
Citrus pith: eat a little citrus pith every day.
Buckwheat: high in rutin, which strengthens vein walls.
Rosemary tea: drink with lemon juice. p155

Warts
Garlic: apply a small amount of crushed garlic to the wart, taking care as it can blister the surrounding skin. p96
Lemon: apply lemon juice or mix peel with crushed garlic. p107

Wasp stings
Vinegar: p180

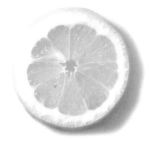

Notes to the text
Recommended reading
Resources
Index

Notes to the text

Full citation given in first reference only, thereafter author and page number; original year of publication in square brackets; place of publication London unless otherwise noted; PubMed references include date and online reference number

Introduction [viii]: Royal Society for the Prevention of Accidents: infocentre@rospa.org [all websites last consulted 14 Jan 2019]; Christopher Hedley & Non Shaw, *Herbal Remedies* (Bath, 2002 [1996]), 6; St Augustine, *On the Good of Marriage* [c. AD 401], 25, http://eng.orthodoxonline.org. **The ingredients [x]:** Cavendish letter: www.peaklandheritage.org.uk; Sophia Baillie: Norfolk Record Office [NRO], BOL 4/7/1–6, 737X1, 1819, unpaginated. **Using kitchen medicines [xii]:** Friedrich von Logau, *Sinngedichte* (c. 1654); Jonathan Swift, *Polite Conversation* (c. 1738); Thomas Edison, in *Newark Advertiser*, 2 Jan 1903 [en.wikiquote.org]; Jill Davies, *The Complete Home Guide to Herbs, Natural Healing and Nutrition* (2003), 3 [www.herbs-hands-healing.co.uk].

ALLSPICE [2–4]: John Ray, *Historia Plantarum* (1693), cited James B McNair, *Spices and Condiments* (Chicago, 1930), 254, biodiversitylibrary.org; *The Oxford Companion to Food*, ed. Alan Davidson (Oxford, 2014), 13; 'official': *The Encyclopedia of Herbs and Herbalism*, ed. Malcolm Stuart (New York, 1979), 239; 'Caribbean stews': Ellen Michaud, *The Healing Kitchen* (Dallas, TX, 2005), 169.

ALMOND [5–7]: Tutankhamun: Jonathan Roberts, *Cabbages & Kings* (2001), 50; William Woodville, *Medical Botany*, 4 vols (1790–3), pl. 183, p507, courtesy of John Innes Foundation Historical Collections, Norwich; John Gerard, *Herball* (1597), quoted Mrs M Grieve, *A Modern Herbal* (1973 [1931]), 24; FFPA: Julia Lawless, *The Encyclopedia of Essential Oils* (Shaftesbury, Dorset, 1992), 41; 'fill the brain': *Hildegard of Bingen's Medicine*, ed. Wighard Strehlow & Gottfried Hertzka, trans. Karin Anderson Strehlow (Santa Fe, NM, 1988), 25; William T Fernie, *Herbal Simples Approved for Modern Uses of Cure* (1914,

[1895]), 20, cited Matthew Wood, *The Earthwise Herbal* (Berkeley, CA, 2008), 85; Dr HCA Vogel, *The Nature Doctor* (Edinburgh, 1990 [1952]), 535; Rose Elliot & Carlo de Paoli, *Kitchen Pharmacy* (New York, 1995 [1991]), 166; AA Gill, *Table Talk* (2007), 75; *J Nutr Sci* 2016 5 e34 [PMC 5048189].

ANISEED, ANISE [8–9]: Leonard Fuchs, *New Kreuterbuch* (1543), quoted Christian Rätsch, *Plants of Love* (Berkeley, CA, 1997), 133; Pliny, quoted Davidson, 23; wedding cake: Mrs Grieve, 42; William Turner, *Herbal*, part 1 (1551), quoted Mrs Grieve, 42; *Solamen intestinorum*: Mrs CF Leyel, *Herbal Delights* (1987 [1937]), 198; Commission E, cited *Herbal Drugs and Phytopharmaceuticals*, ed. Norman Grainger Bisset & Max Wichtl, 2nd edn (Stuttgart/Boca Raton, FL, 2001 [1994]), 74; 'hard coughs': Wood, *Earthwise*, 383; Gerard, quoted KV Smith, *The Illustrated Earth Garden Herbal* (1979 [1978]), 39; John Parkinson, *Theatrum Botanicum* (1640), 911; Sir John Harington, *The Englishmans Doctor* (1607), quoted KV Smith, 39; Hedley & Shaw, 75.

APPLE [10–13]: 'apple a day', apple dumplings: Roy Vickery, *Dictionary of Plant Lore* (Oxford, 1997 [1995]), 12; Michael Pollan, *The Botany of Desire* (2002), 18, 22; waxing, 44lb: Michaud, 38, usapple.org, 2014; Fernie, quoted Wood, *Earthwise*, 413; Mrs Grieve, 46; Jane Austen, letter to Cassandra [sister], 17 October 1815; Jean Palaiseul, *Grandmother's Secrets*, trans. Pamela Swinglehurst (1976 [1972]), 31; 'Wildman' Steve Brill with Evelyn Dean, *Identifying and Harvesting Edible and Medicinal Plants* (New York, 1994), 151–2, 153; 'dentist': Mrs Leyel, *Herbal Delights*, 106; Bircher-Benner, lanolin: Palaiseul, 33; Henry Thoreau, 'Wild Apples', *Atlantic Monthly*, 1862, 59, www.manybooks.net; Roberts, 38

ARROWROOT [14–15]: Napoleon:

MS Palaniswami & Shirly Raichal Anil, *Tuber & Root Crops* (New Delhi, 2008), 25; name: Mrs Grieve, 57; *Kenya Settlers' Cookery Book and Household Guide*, 12th edn (Nairobi, 1957), 134–5.

BANANA [16–17]: genes: www.kew.org/ksheets/banana.html; US data: www.fao.org and www.seeker.com; UK data: Robin McKie, *The Observer*, 30 June 2002.

BARLEY [18–21]: David Hoffmann, *Medical Herbalism* (Rochester, VT, 2003), 378; 'booze': Franz G Meussdoerffer, 'A Comprehensive History of Beer Brewing', in *A Handbook of Brewing*, ed. Dr Hans Michael Esslinger (Mannheim, Germany, 2009), 7; Hildegard, 111; William Meyrick, *The New Family Herbal* (Birmingham, 1789), 28; barley water: campaignlive.co.uk, 27 Jun 2014; in the kitchen: Davidson, 64–5; and cholesterol: *Eur J Clin Nutr*, Nov 2016 [PMID 27273067].

BASIL [21–25]: *pesto, soupe au pistou*: Palaiseul, 45; John Hill, *The Family Herbal* (Bungay, Suffolk, 1812), 26; useful herb: Joe Nasr, lecture notes, April 2002; *basilicus*: Deni Bown, *Herbal* (2001), 184; Wood, *Earthwise*, 361; William Turner, *Herbal*, parts 1 and 2 (1568), quoted KV Smith, 45; John Parkinson, *Paradisi in Sole: Paradisus Terrestris* (1976 [1629]), 450; Meyrick, 30; Sebastian Pole, *Ayurvedic Medicine* (Amsterdam, 2006), 280; Gerard, quoted KV Smith, 45; David Winston & Steven Maimes, *Adaptogens* (Rochester, VT, 2007), 167–71.

BEETROOT, RED BEET [26–27]: Gerard, *Herball*, Marcus Woodward edn (1994), 68–9; Hill, 32; *J Int Sports Nutri* v15, 2018 [PMC 5756374]; Geoffrey Grigson, *The Englishman's Flora* (1975 [1958]), 106; Penelope Ody, *Essential Guide to Natural Home Remedies* (2002 [1997]), 111.

BICARBONATE OF SODA, BAKING SODA [28–31]: Tabitha Tickletooth [pseud. of Charles Selby], *The Dinner Question* (1860), quoted Davidson, 79 Margaret Briggs, *Bicarbonate of Soda* (Edinburgh, 2007), 21; Ben Charles Harris, *Kitchen Medicines* (New York, 1968 [1961]), 144; 'corpse reviver': Tim Noakes, *Lore of Running* (Cape Town, 1985), 304.

BLUEBERRY [32–33]: Thoreau, quoted *Wild Fruits*, ed. Bradley P Dean (New York, 2000), 52; sales in Britain: *Food Lovers' Guide*, suppl. *The Times* (Autumn 2009), 24, and www.sefari. scot; Nutrient Data Laboratory, USDA, http://ndb.nal.usda.gov; ars.usda.gov.

BUTTER & GHEE [34–37]: milk allergies: Christine Herbert, pers. comm., 20 Apr 2010; Davidson, 121–2 (butter), 347 (ghee); Vasant Lad, *Complete Book of Ayurvedic Home Remedies* (New York, 1999), 286.

CABBAGE [38–41]: Mrs CF Leyel, *Cinquefoil* (1957), 33; Boerhaave syrup: Palaiseul, 69; Parkinson, *Paradisi*, 505; John Evelyn, *Acetaria: A Discourse on Sallets* (Brooklyn, NY, 1937 [1699]), 10; Pliny, *The Natural History*, ed. John Bostock & HT Riley (1855), 20: 33, www.questia.com; Parkinson, *Paradisi*, 505; Dr Cheney: Harris, 43; Dr Valnet: Elliot & De Paoli, 94; Valentine: Vickery, 57; James Duke, *The Green Pharmacy* (Emmaus, PA, 1997), 340.

CARDAMOM, ELACHI [42–45]: top table: Carol Ann Rinzler, *Herbs, Spices and Condiments* (New York, 1990), 38; 'queen of spices': HK Bakhru, *Herbs that Heal* (New Delhi, 1990), 52; Dr Torrebiarte, quoted Larry Luxner, *Saudi Aramco World* 48/2 (1997), 30; Raffles: quoted IH Burkhill, *A Dictionary of the Economic Products of the Malay Peninsula*, 2 vols (1935), I, 913; David Frawley & Vasant Lad, *The Yoga of Herbs*, 2nd edn (Twin Lakes, WI, 2001 [1986]), 109; Pole, 151; Duke, 76.

CARROT [46–47]: Richard Gardiner, quoted Jean Carper, *Foods that Heal* (New York, 1988), 156; Duke, 400;

Hindu Kush: Roberts, 153; 'carrot factor': Carper, 77.

CELERY [48–49]: Meyrick, 89; *selinon*: Davidson, 149; Mme de Pompadour: Charles Connell, *Aphrodisiacs in Your Garden* (1965), 35; *British Herbal Pharmacopoeia 1996* (1996), 56; Andrew Chevallier, *Herbal Remedies* (2007), 69.

CHILLI/CAYENNE PEPPER [50–54]: Columbus: quoted Jack Turner, *Spice: The History of a Temptation* (2005), 12; Chris Kilham, *Psyche Delicacies* (Emmaus, PA, 2001), 87ff; Hedley & Shaw, 61; Matthew Wood, *The Book of Herbal Wisdom* (Berkeley, CA, 1997), 188; chilli con-fusion: Roberts, 182–3; *King's American Dispensatory*, ed. Harvey Wickes Felter & John Uri Lloyd (1898), www.henriettes-herb. com; Dr John R Christopher, *School of Natural Healing* (Springville, UT, 1996 [1976]), 447.

CHOCOLATE [54–57]: Moctezuma: quoted Stuart Lee Allen, *In the Devil's Garden* (Edinburgh, 2002), 32ff; www. cadbury.co.uk; 'mouthfeel': Craig Sams & Josephine Fairley, *Sweet Dreams* (2008), 57; mayoclinic.org; Sams & Fairley, 47; Jim McDonald, www. herb@lists.ibiblio.org, 2009.

CINNAMON [58–61]: Nero: www. theepicentre.com; Sethos I: quoted Lisa Maniche, *An Egyptian Herbal* (1989), 91; St Augustine: quoted Turner, 249; Michaud, 175; Bede: quoted Turner, 183; posset: Turner, 216.

CLOVES [62–64]: Chinese emperor: Stuart, 269; nail: Turner, xxxv; Tom Stobart (ed.), *The Cook's Encyclopaedia* (1980), cited in Davidson, 198; Hedley & Shaw, 68; Mrs Grieve, 208.

COCONUT [65–67]: 'boons': Monisha Bharadwaj, *The Indian Kitchen* (1996), 114; 'most useful': Harris, 59–60 and Davidson, 199, 201; Burkhill, I, 598.

COFFEE [68–71]: Sir Thomas Herbert: quoted Sybil Kapoor, *Taste* (2003), 87; Pope Clement VIII: William H Ukers, *All About Coffee* (New York, 1922), 26, babel.hathitrust.org; Yemeni Sufis:

Claudia Roden, *A Book of Middle Eastern Food* (1970 [1968]), 456; Hill, 84; Paul Bergner, *Med Herbalism: A Journal for the Clinical Practitioner* 16/1 (2009), 1–14; Kapoor, 87; R Bentley & H Trimen, *Medicinal Plants*, 4 vols (1880), III, 144.

CORIANDER, CILANTRO [72–75]: manna: Bharadwaj, 34; Sir Hugh Plat, *Delights for Ladies* (1609), quoted Miranda Seymour, *A Brief History of Thyme* (2002), 37; Pliny's name: Seymour, 38; garnish: Bharadwaj, 34; Stuart, 179; Parkinson, *Theatrum*, 918; freshener: Duke, 77; William Salmon, *The New London Dispensatory* (1696), www.historicfood.com; Pole, 165.

CORN, MAIZE [76–79]: FAO data, faostat.fao.org; Gerard, 26 [Woodward edn]; pellagra: www.encyclopedia. com; *British Herbal Pharmacopoeia 1996*, 64; Duke, 51; Gill, 177.

CRANBERRY [80–81]: 'crane-berry': Brill & Dean, 224; Pilgrim Fathers, sorting machines: Davidson, 227–8; 'receptor blockade': Carper, 81, 180–2; trials: Amanda Ursell, *The Times*, 27 July 2009; health benefits overview: *J Food Sci*, 9 Jan 2018 [PMID 29315597]; Chevallier, *Herbal Remedies*, 236.

CUMIN [82–84]: Pliny: quoted Davidson, 233; Hill, 103; Pole, 167; George VI: Florence Ranson, *British Herbs* (1949), 156; Spenser: quoted Mrs Leyel, *Herbal Delights*, 215; caraway: Mrs Grieve, 158; illustration from Parkinson, *Theatrum*, 887.

DILL [85–87]: Hoffmann, 527; Thomas Jefferson, c. 1785: quoted on pickle websites; 'meetin' seed': Susan Lavender & Anna Franklin, *Herb Craft* (Chieveley, Berks, 1996), 200; Pickle Packers International, www. ilovepickles.org; Duke, 43; carvone: Rintzler, 67; Parkinson, *Paradisi*, 494.

FENNEL [88–91]: Indian names: Pole, 175; Prometheus: Davidson, 303; Anglo-Saxon sacred herbs: the others are mugwort, plantain, watercress, atherlothe [possibly betony or viper's bugloss], chamomile, nettle, crab apple and chervil; Myddfai: quoted KV Smith, 71; Harington, *The Englishmans Doctor* (1607), 104–5; Hildegard: quoted Hedley & Shaw, 20; Abbé Kneipp: quoted Palaiseul, 118.

FENUGREEK [92–93]: ballad of Lydia Pinkham: eg http://sniff.numachi.com; Parkinson, *Theatrum*, 1097; 'Greek hay': Stuart, 274; Lydia Pinkham: Duke, 88; sprouts: Julian Barker, *The Medicinal Flora of Britain and Northwestern Europe* (West Wickham, Kent, 2001), 156 (p203); Parkinson, *Theatrum*, 1097; diabetes: Duke, 163.

FIGS [94–95]: trees in Bible, Hezekiah: Palaiseul, 119; Ebers MS: Ody, 124; John Pechey, *The Compleat Herbal of Physical Plants*, 2nd edn (1707), 91; Meyrick, 169; Fernie, 197; natron remedy: Maniche, 103; Pechey, 91; Pliny: quoted Carper, 188; Parkinson, *Theatrum*, 1495.

GARLIC [96–99]: Stephen Harrod Buhner, *Herbal Antibiotics* (North Adams, MA, 1999), 33; Aristophanes: quoted Stuart Lee Allen, 245; pyramids: Bharadwaj, 112; Harrington: modernised from *The Englishmans Doctor* by Michael T Murray, *The Healing Power of Herbs*, 2nd edn (Roseville, CA, 1995 [1992]), 122 [Harington was himself adapting an older text, the twelfth-century *Regimen Sanitatis Salernitatum*]; Ian Hemphill, *The Spice and Herb Bible*, 2nd edn (Toronto, 2006 [2000]), 271; Evelyn, 18; 'four thieves', see eg Victoria Renoux, *For the Love of Garlic* (New York, 2005), 19, http://books.google.com.

GINGER [100–103]: Francis Beaumont & John Fletcher, *The Knight of the Burning Pestle* (1609), I.4 [probably borrowed from an earlier drinking song]; Pole, 183; Laurel Dewey, *The Humorous Herbalist* (East Canaan, CT, 1996), 81–2.

HONEY [104–106]: botulism caution: Paul Pitchford, *Healing with Whole Foods* (Berkeley, CA, 1993), 258; Muslim story: KV Smith, 49; rock painting, Sumerian tablets: Davidson, 384; milk and honey: Exodus, 3.8;

Hippocrates: Juliette de Baïracli Levy, *The Complete Herbal Book of the Dog* (1971), 207; Shakespeare, *Henry IV, Part One* (1597), 3.2; James Green, *The Herbal Medicine-Maker's Handbook* (Berkeley, CA, 2000), 244; Jonathan Swift, *The Battle of the Books* (1704); mead: NRO, Receipt Book, MC43/6, unpaginated, undated.

LEMON [107–109]: names: Stuart, 175; Louis XIV's court: Roberts, 100; Sydney Smith: quoted Lady Holland, *A Memoir of the Reverend Sydney Smith*, 2 vols (New York, 1855), I, 262; Mrs Grieve, 475; Peter Holmes, *The Energetics of Western Herbs*, 2nd edn, 2 vols (Berkeley, CA, 1993 [1989]), II, 594; alkalising: Andrew Chevallier, *Encyclopedia of Herbal Medicine* (2016 [1996]), 81; Bentley & Trimen, I, 54; earliest lemonade recipe: www.cliffordawright.com.

MUSHROOMS [110–111]: Tobias Venner, *Via Recta ad Vitam Longam* (1620), quoted Georges M Halpern, *Healing Mushrooms* (New York, 2007), 11; Peter Jordan & Steven Wheeler, *The Ultimate Mushroom Book* (1995), 9; 2009 Chinese study: Min Zhang et al, *Int J Cancer*, 15 Mar 2009 [PMID 19048616]; button mushrooms: Zhihong Ren et al., *J Nutr* 138 (Mar 2008), 544–50; Thomas Bartram, *Bartram's Encyclopedia of Herbal Medicine* (1995), 390 [quoting Paul Callinan]; Christopher Hobbs, lecture, HerbFest, Worcester, UK, 1 Aug 2009.

MUSTARD [112–114]: Mrs Clements: Mrs Grieve, 568; 'a contemporary': Richard Bradley, *The Country Housewife and Lady's Director* (1980 [1736]), 37; mustard cf. pepper: Plochman website: www.plochman.com; Meyrick, 336; Green, 283; FN Howes, *A Dictionary of Useful and Everyday Plants* (1973), 169; chilblains remedy: NRO, HMN4/7/4: Household recipes, 18th century.

NUTMEG & MACE [115–117]: history: Giles Milton, *Nathaniel's Nutmeg* (1999), 17, 373; Pechey, 309; Christine Herbert, *Nature's Path 8/2* (Summer 2009), 8–11; Meyrick, 350; Peter Piper: www.bonappetit.com.

OATS [118–121]: 'manured oates', illus in Parkinson, *Theatrum*, 1134; oats to Britain: Davidson, 565; horses: Francesco Bianchini et al., *The Complete Book of Fruits and Vegetables*, trans. Italia & Alberto Mancinelli (New York, 1973), 18; Irish saying: Joanne Asala, *Celtic Folklore Cooking* (Woodbury, MN, 2005 [1998]), 108; Burns, 'The Cotter's Saturday Night' (1786), quoted GW Lockhart, *The Scots and Their Oats*, 2nd edn (Edinburgh, 1997 [1983]), 31; Fergusson, 'The Farmer's Ingle' (1771), quoted Lockhart, 31; Johnson, *Dictionary of the English Language* (1755), www.bl.uk/learning; Mrs Leyel, *Hearts-Ease: Herbs for the Heart* (1949), 288; no famine: Holmes, I, 404; Pechey, 175; Abbé Kneipp: quoted Palaiseul, 228; Thomas Tryon, *The Good House-wife Made a Doctor*, 2nd edn (1692), 270; Plat, 90; and cholesterol: *Br J Nutr*, Oct 2016 [PMID 27724985]; US herbalism, eg Wood, *Earthwise*, 124; Dr Vogel, 371; Carper, 240.

OLIVE [122–125]: Roman health cliché: *Encyclopedia Britannica*, 10th edn (1902), www.1902encyclopedia.com; virgin oil: La Vialla, Tuscany, www.lavialla.it; first fruits: Roberts, 109; superior oil: Barker, 261 (p323); atherosclerosis: *Eur J Nutr*, Aug 2012 [PMID 22872323]; 'diet for the skin': www.olivellaline.com; olive leaves: Wood, *Earthwise*, 365; lubricates: Wood, *Earthwise*, 364; Barker, 261 (p323).

ONION [126–129]: lilies of the field: Matthew 6.29; Egypt: Herodotus, *Histories*, trans. Robin Waterfield (Oxford, 2008), book 2.125 (p145), www.books.google.co.uk, Evelyn, 32; Jean Anthelme Brillat-Savarin (1755–1826) supposedly said this [and also 'most of the food allergies die under garlic and onion']; umami: Kapoor, 10, 11; 64mt: FAO, 2005 data; Libya: www.onions-usa.org; Jonathan Swift, 'Verses Made for Fruit Women' (c. 1720): www.online-literature.com; Martial, *Epigrams* Book X, no. XVII: www.archive.org; within oral tradition: Gabrielle Hatfield, *Country Remedies* (Woodbridge, Suffolk, 1994), 28–30; *Perfumed Garden*, trans. Sir Richard Burton (1886); medieval image: Carol

Belanger Grafton, *Medieval Herb, Plant and Flower Illustrations* (New York, 1997 [CD-ROM, 2004], image 102; 1952 saying: Vickery, 267; Richo Cech, *Making Plant Medicine* (Williams, OR, 2000), 92–3; English newspaper: NRO, MC43/8, undated; poultice: Cech, 96; Baillie: Sophia Baillie, Recipe Book, 1819, NRO, BOL 4/19, 741X5; onion peel extract and lipid profile, *Nutr Res Pract*, Oct 2013 [PMID 24133616].

ORANGE [130–132]: 'orange' name: Bianchini, 182; FCOJ: Roberts, 102; Eau-de-Cologne: Sarah Garland, *The Herb and Spice Book* (1979), 249; Parkinson, *Theatrum*, 1509; Hill, 250; Wood, *Earthwise*, 196.

OREGANO & MARJORAM [133–135]: comparison: Davidson, 479–80, 557 and Hemphill, 360–4; oregano by 'flavour': Arthur Tucker & Michael Macciarello, in *Spices, Herbs and Edible Fungi*, ed. G. Charalambous (Amsterdam, 1994), 439–56, cited Davidson, 567; 'joy of the mountain', KV Smith, 105 and Audrey Wynne Hatfield, *Pleasures of Herbs* (1964), 89; Parkinson, *Paradisi*, 453; Shakespeare, *All's Well That Ends Well* (1601–8), 4.5; Nicholas Culpeper, *The English Physician Enlarged* (1995 [1653]), 160; Holmes, II, 541; Hill, 218, 217; John Nott, *The Cook's and Confectioner's Dictionary* (1723), 25, quoted KV Smith, 94 and www.books.google.co.uk.

PARSLEY [136–139]: name: Mrs Grieve, 611; 'in need of parsley': TF Thiselton-Dyer, *The Folk-Lore of Plants* (1994 [1889]), 140; superstitions: Palaiseul, 238; popularity, *persillade*: Davidson, 596; cultivars: Bown, 207; Thomas Coghan, *The Haven of Health* (1584), quoted KV Smith, 106; Wood, *Earthwise*, 379; 'useful umbellifers': Clive Stace, *Field Flora of the British Isles* (Cambridge, 1999), 347; *British Herbal Pharmacopoeia 1996*, 148; Dr Christopher, 268; illustration from Gerard, *Herball*, CD-ROM & Book, Dover Electronic Clip Art edn (Mineola, NY, 2005), image 181 (p40).

PEPPER [140–144]: 'king of spices': Hemphill, 396; Vasco da Gama: Stuart,

241; Pliny, *Natural History* 12.14, quoted Ody, *Natural Home Remedies*, 94–5; Edward Gibbon, *The History of the Decline and Fall of the Roman Empire* (1776–88), ch. XXX, n79 ['the improvement of trade and navigation has multiplied the quantity [of pepper] and reduced the price'], www.fullbooks.com; Pliny, in Ody, *Natural Home Remedies*, 95; Evelyn, 34; John Chamberlayne, *A Family-Herbal* (1689), 121; 'robust oiliness': Hemphill, 405; 'cook pathogens': Pole, 237; Hill, 260.

PINEAPPLE [144–145]: Sir Walter Raleigh, *Discovery of Guiana* (1595), 58: www.bartleby.com; Elliot & De Paoli (1991), 196; bromelain: Burkhill, I, 152; boxers' bruises: Duke, 108; wrinkles: Duke, 461; *nana*: Davidson, 626–7; folk remedy: Bartram, 339.

POPPY SEED [146–147]: O. Phelps Brown, *The Complete Herbalist* (1907), 131.

PUMPKIN [148–149]: Hill, 274; *Dispensatory of the United States*, ed. Joseph P. Remington, Horatio Wood et al. (1918), www.henriettes-herb.com [under *Pepo*]; Bisset & Wichtl, 171; BPH, Dr Mongenay: Duke, 367–70; tapeworm: Bartram, 415–16.

RICE [150–151]: Davidson, 681–3; Palaiseul, 271; plant-based 'milks': *J Food Sci Tech*, Sept 2016 [PMID 27777447].

ROSEMARY [152–155]: Holmes, I, 338; William Langham, *The Garden of Health* (1597), quoted KV Smith, 111; Evelyn, 39; 'dew of the sea': Stuart, 254 and Seymour, 96; exam time: Barbara Hey, *A Celebration of Herbs for the South African Garden & Home* (Cape Town, 1992), 62; Robert Herrick (nd), quoted Audrey Wynne Hatfield, 107; *Banckes' Herbal*, quoted Agnes Arber, *Herbals, Their Origin and Evolution* (Cambridge, 1912), 39; Walther Ryff, quoted Holmes, I, 338; Queen of Hungary water: Palaiseul, 274; de Baïracli Levy, 123; acetylcholine and Alzheimer's: *Evid Based Comp Alt Med*, Jan 2016 [PMID 26941822]; Pechey, 206; Don Quixote: cited Seymour, 97.

SAGE [156–159]: 'saviour': Audrey Wynne Hatfield, 113; 'a man die': *Regimen*, 6; Coghan, *Haven* (1584), quoted KV Smith, 118; Harington (1607), quoted KV Smith, 118; China/Dutch trade-off: Hemphill, 449; Boston Tea Party: Seymour, 104; Bradley, 92; Mrs Leathe, NRO, BOL 2/167, 740X7, undated, unpaginated; illustration from Gerard, *Herball*, CD-ROM & Book, image 127 (p28); Walafrid Strabo (c. AD 840), quoted KV Smith, 118; Ranson, 182; Maria Treben, *Health through God's Pharmacy* (Steyr, Austria, 1982), 37; Wood, *Earthwise*, 450; Penelope Ody, *Herbs for First Aid* (Los Angeles, CA, 1999), 36; Margaret Roberts, *Margaret Roberts' Book of Herbs* (Bergvlei, South Africa, 1983), 14.

SALT [160–163]: Elizabeth David, *Spices, Salt and Aromatics in the English Kitchen* (2000 [1970]), 49; salt of the earth: Matthew 5.13; 'worth his salt': also a Roman soldier not earning his wage; Pitchford, 157; Evelyn, 64; Pitchford, 156; 'salt of youth': Shakespeare, *The Merry Wives of Windsor* (1602), 2.3; 'grain of salt' may be from Pliny, who records that a little salt [and a lot of rue] was an antidote to poison; 'spoonful of sugar' is a song from *Mary Poppins* (1964).

STAR ANISE [164–165]: Stuart, 206; illustration from Bentley & Trimen, III, 217, courtesy of John Innes Foundation Historical Collections, Norwich; Wood, *Earthwise*, 301; FDA advisory, 10 Sept 2003, www.fda.gov; Tamiflu: www.tamiflu.com and National Public Radio (US), 18 May 2009, www.npr.org.

SUGAR [166–167]: 'pure, white and deadly': title of book by nutritionist John Yudkin (1988 [1972]); Chamberlayne, 219.

TEA [168–172]: Thomas Garway (1658): quoted Francis Leggett & Co, *Tea from the Tea-garden to the Tea Cup* (New York, 1900), www.henriettes-herb.com; Sydney Smith: quoted Lady Holland, I, 337; 'bread and water': source claimed to be *Oakland Tribune*, 13 May 1903; Alice Walker websites cite the phrase but give no exact reference; Buddha story: Bown, 66; 'antioxidant punch': Barbara Griggs, *Helpful Herbs* (Oxford, 2008), 202; Sir Kenelm Digby, *The Closet of the Eminently Learned Sir Kenelm Digby Knight Opened 1669*, quoted David, 246; EGCG: www.alczap.thorne.com (2.14); illustration from Bentley & Trimen, I, 35, courtesy of John Innes Foundation Historical Collections, Norwich; Mrs Grieve, 793; Typhoo, PG Tips: Reader's Digest, *Foods that Harm, Foods that Heal* (1996), 72; Mongolian meal: Henry C Lu, *Chinese Natural Cures* (New York, 1994), 304; tea bags: Harris, 154; William Cobbett, *Cottage Economy* (1833), 19, www.books.google.co.uk; Chevallier, *Herbal Remedies*, 88; caffeine comparison: *Foods that Harm*, 72.

THYME [173–175]: *thumon*: Seymour, 116; fumigation: Hedley & Shaw, 78 and Mrs Grieve, 809; Holmes, I, 229; Culpeper, 258; Margaret Roberts, 23; Francis Bacon, 'On Gardens' (1625), archive.ub.uni-heidelberg.de; illustration from Gerard, *Herball*, CD-ROM & Book, image 80 (p18); Holmes, I, 229; Wood, *Earthwise*, 484.

TURMERIC [176–179]: Marco Polo: Davidson, 838; Parkinson, *Theatrum*, 1584; Indian BandAid™: *Wall Street Journal*, 30 Aug 2005, online.wsj.com/article; Duke, 314; Pole, 282; H. Hatcher et al., *Cell Mol Life Sci* 65/11 (2008), 1631–52 [PMID 18324353]; Joe & Teresa Graedon, *Best Choices from the People's Pharmacy* (New York, 2007), 121–3, 615; Mrs Grieve, 823; curcumin: Chevallier, *Encyclopedia*, 90; 'solid gold': BB Aggarwal et al., *Adv. Exp. Med. Biol.* 595 (2007), 1–75 [PMID 17569205].

VINEGAR [180–182]: 'vin aigre': Chamberlayne, 210; maturing: Davidson, 828; Graedon & Graedon, 620; Parkinson, *Theatrum*, 1558; LP Elwell-Sutton, *Persian Proverbs* (1954), 28; Chamberlayne, 211, 212; Dr James Malone recipe ['highly recommended' added to original], NRO, MC 43/8, undated, unpaginated.

WATER [183–185]: Karen C Uphoff, *Botanical Body Care* (Fort Bragg, CA, 2007), 65, 102, 203–10; Sylvia Plath, *The Bell Jar* (1963), quoted Griggs, 195; RW Clark, *JBS: The Life and Work of J.B.S. Haldane* (Oxford, 1984); 'our water world': *Foods that Harm*, 372–5.

Yogurt [186–188]: *lebne*: Davidson, 886; lactose intolerance: Davidson, 454; NHS trials: eg 4 Feb 2008, BBC, www.news.bbc.co.uk; also thelancet.com 382: 9900, 1249–57, 12 Oct 2013.

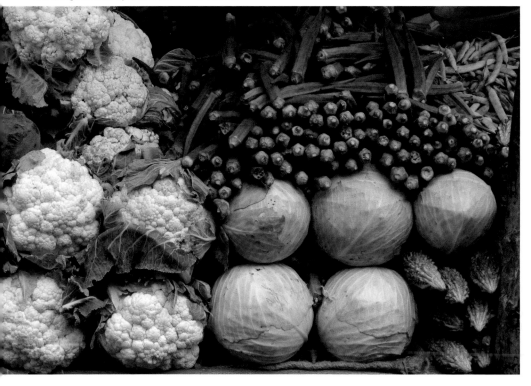

Recommended reading

Bartram, Thomas. *Bartram's Encyclopedia of Herbal Medicine.* London, 1998 (1995)

Bharadwaj, Monisha. *The Indian Kitchen.* London, 1998 (1996)

Cech, Richo. *Making Plant Medicine.* Williams, OR, 2000

Chevallier, Andrew. *Encyclopedia of Herbal Medicine*, 3rd edn. London, 2016 (1996)
—— *Herbal Remedies.* London, 2007

David, Elizabeth. *Spices, Salt and Aromatics in the English Kitchen.* London, 2000 (1970)

Davidson, Alan (ed.). *The Oxford Companion to Food*, 3rd edn (ed. Tom Jaine). Oxford, 2014 (1999)

Duke, James A. *The Green Pharmacy.* Emmaus, PA, 1997

Elliot, Rose & De Paoli, Carlo. *Kitchen Pharmacy: How to Make Your Own Remedies.* New York, 1995 (1991)

Green, James. *The Herbal Medicine-Maker's Handbook: A Home Manual.* Berkeley, CA, 2002

Griggs, Barbara. *Helpful Herbs for Health and Beauty.* Oxford, 2008

Grieve, Mrs M. *A Modern Herbal.* London, 1998 (1931); online at www.botanical.com

Harris, Ben Charles. *Kitchen Medicines.* New York, 1968 (1961)

Hedley, Christopher & Shaw, Non. *Herbal Remedies: A Practical Beginner's Guide to Making Effective Remedies in the Kitchen.* Bath, 2002 (1996)

Hemphill, Ian. *The Spice and Herb Bible*, 2nd edn. Toronto, 2006 (2002)

Holmes, Peter. *The Energetics of Western Herbs: A Materia Medica Integrating Western and Oriental Herbal Medicine Traditions*, 2nd edn, 2 vols. Berkeley, CA, 1993 (1989)

Lad, Usha & Lad, Vasant. *Ayurvedic Cooking for Self-Healing*, 2nd edn. Albuquerque, NM, 1997 (1994)

Michaud, Ellen. *The Healing Kitchen.* Dallas, TX, 2005

Ody, Penelope. *Herbs for First Aid: Simple Home Remedies for Minor Ailments and Injuries.* Los Angeles, CA, 1999
_____ *Essential Guide to Natural Home Remedies.* London, 2002

Palaiseul, Jean. *Grandmother's Secrets: Her Green Guide to Health from Plants.* Trans. Pamela Swinglehurst. London, 1973 (1972)

Pinnock, Dale. *Medicinal Cookery: How You Can Benefit from Nature's Edible Pharmacy.* London, 2011

Pitchford, Paul. *Healing with Whole Foods: Oriental Traditions and Modern Nutrition.* Berkeley, CA, 1993

Pole, Sebastian. *Ayurvedic Medicine: The Principles of Traditional Practice.* Amsterdam, 2006

Rinzler, Carol Ann. *The Complete Book of Herbs, Spices and Condiments: From Garden to Kitchen to Medicine Chest.* New York, 1980

Roberts, Margaret. *Healing Foods.* Pretoria, South Africa, 2011.

Stuart, Malcolm (ed.). *The Encyclopedia of Herbs and Herbalism.* New York, 1979

Turner, Jack. *Spice: The History of a Temptation.* London, 2005

William, Anthony. *Medical Medium Life-Changing Foods.* London, 2016

Wong, James. *Grow Your Own Drugs: Easy Recipes for Natural Remedies and Beauty Fixes.* London, 2009
_____ *James Wong's Homegrown Revolution.* London, 2012

Wood, Matthew. *The Earthwise Herbal: A Complete Guide to Old World Medicinal Plants.* Berkeley, CA, 2008

Resources

Finding a herbal practitioner

Kitchen medicine is all about healing yourself, but there will be times when you may need the advice of a qualified herbalist. To find a practitioner near you, contact the (British) professional associations listed below. Complementary therapy clinics in your area may have herbalists working there, and you can ask your local health food store to make a recommendation.

Association of Master Herbalists (AMH)
www.associationofmasterherbalists.co.uk

College of Practitioners of Phytotherapy (CPP)
01323 484 353
www.thecpp.uk

The International Register of Consultant Herbalists and Homoeopaths (IRCH)
info@irch.org.uk
www.irch.org

National Institute of Medical Herbalists (NIMH)
01392 426 022
www.nimh.org.uk

Unified Register of Herbal Practitioners (URHP)
7539 528857
www.urhp.com

Suppliers

You can find most of what you need for our style of kitchen medicine in grocery, kitchen and hardware stores. Here are a few mail order companies who carry harder-to-source materials.

Avicenna
01570 471 000
avicenna@clara.co.uk
Mail order: aromatic waters, creams, organically grown herbs.

G Baldwin & Co
020 7703 5550
www.baldwins.co.uk
Mail order and shop: brown glass bottles, lanolin, beeswax; also dried herbs, essential oils.

Fattoria La Vialla
www.lavialla.it
0039 0575 477720
Mail order: organic/biodynamic farm in Tuscany with a beautiful catalogue; the food is lovely.

Herbs, Hands, Healing
01379 608 201
www.herbs-hands-healing.co.uk
Mail order: culinary herbs and medicinal herbal products, with a herbalist's kitchen range.

Lakeland Ltd
01539 488 100
www.lakeland.co.uk
Mail order and stores: jam- and jelly-making supplies, kitchen equipment.

Neals Yard Remedies
10747 834698
www.nealsyardremedies.com
Mail order and shops: beeswax, lanolin, brown glass bottles; also herbs and body care.

Pukka Herbs
0845 375 1744
www.pukkaherbs.com
Mail order, many products (eg herb teas) available in stores: organically grown spices and herbs, Ayurvedic books.

The London Teapot Company
0845 230 4566
www.chatsford.com
Mail order, manufacturer: Chatsford teapots with removable strainers for loose teas.

Tree Harvest
01297 552 977
www.tree-harvest.com
Mail order: non-timber forest products – nuts, seeds, berries, oils, herbs and spices.

World of Spice
01277 633303
worldofspice.co.uk
Mail order: online shop for spices, herbs, wax, jars, etc.

Plant information

The Herb Society
www.herbsociety.org.uk
An educational charity that promotes interest in all aspects of herbs, including cookery, medicine, dyeing and gardening; publishes *Herbs* magazine.

Index

The authors

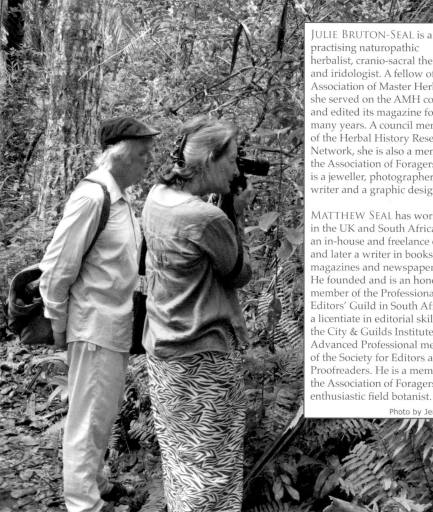

JULIE BRUTON-SEAL is a practising naturopathic herbalist, cranio-sacral therapist and iridologist. A fellow of the Association of Master Herbalists, she served on the AMH council and edited its magazine for many years. A council member of the Herbal History Research Network, she is also a member of the Association of Foragers. She is a jeweller, photographer, artist, writer and a graphic designer.

MATTHEW SEAL has worked in the UK and South Africa as an in-house and freelance editor and later a writer in books, magazines and newspapers. He founded and is an honorary member of the Professional Editors' Guild in South Africa, is a licentiate in editorial skills of the City & Guilds Institute and an Advanced Professional member of the Society for Editors and Proofreaders. He is a member of the Association of Foragers and an enthusiastic field botanist.

Photo by Jen Bartlett

Other books by Julie and Matthew:
Backyard Medicine: Harvest and Make Your Own Herbal Remedies; Backyard Medicine for All: A Guide to Home-Grown Herbal Remedies; The Herbalist's Bible: John Parkinson's Lost Classic Rediscovered; Make Your Own Aphrodisiacs.

For workshops, courses and other information, see their website: www.hedgerowmedicine.com